OXFORD MEDICAL PUBLICATIONS

Unplanned Pregnancy: your choices

D0864364

Unplanned pregnancy: your choices

A practical guide to accidental pregnancy

ANN FUREDI

Director, Birth Control Trust, London and Freelance Medical Journalist

Oxford   Toronto   Melbourne

OXFORD UNIVERSITY PRESS

1996

Oxford University Press, Walton Street, Oxford OX2 6DP

Oxford   New York
Athens   Auckland   Bangkok   Bombay
Calcutta   Cape Town   Dar es Salaam   Delhi
Florence   Hong Kong   Istanbul   Karachi
Kuala Lumpur   Madras   Madrid   Melbourne
Mexico City   Nairobi   Paris   Singapore
Taipei   Tokyo   Toronto

and associated companies in
Berlin   Ibadan

Oxford is a trade mark of Oxford University Press

Published in the United States by Oxford University Press Inc., New York

A catalogue record for this book is available from the British Library

Library of Congress Cataloging in Publication Data
(Data available)

ISBN 0 19 262445 8

Typeset by Footnote Graphics, Warminster

Printed in Great Britain by
Biddles Ltd
Guildford & King's Lynn

Acknowledgements

Over many years of writing on unplanned pregnancy I have spoken with numerous women who have shared their hopes, worries, and fears and were happy to 'go on the record'. I am deeply grateful to you all.

Very special thanks to David Paintin FRCOG and Dilys Cossey OBE who have provided inspiration and advice and allowed me to plunder their knowledge and experience; to the information department of the Family Planning Association, especially Toni Belfield, Jane Urwin, and Margaret McGovern who allowed me to make unreasonable demands on their time and patience; to Alison Hadley of Brook Advisory Centres for being the final word on the needs and concerns of young people; to Amanda Callaghan and David Nolan, friends and colleagues at Birth Control Trust, who have exceeded their own briefs so as to allow me to extend mine; and finally, to my partner Frank Furedi who makes everything possible.

Introduction

'Every month, on the day my period is due to start, I'm nervous in case it doesn't. It's just the way I am. I've felt like this from the first time I had sex. Even if I know in my mind I couldn't be pregnant because, for some reason, I hardly had sex at all, I still get a tense feeling in my stomach if my period hasn't started by the time I leave work on the day it's due.'

'It was late once, and for two days I couldn't concentrate on anything. All I could think about was whether my body felt like it usually did before a period. In the end I didn't know whether I really had backache in the usual way or whether it was just wishful thinking.'

'My period was only four days late, but I had done three pregnancy tests by the time it started. Each one was negative but I had to keep checking, just to reassure myself.'

'Since I started having sex when I was 16, the only months when I haven't worried about [being pregnant] are those when I haven't had sex. I keep telling myself that I must be neurotic. I'm 28 now—and for all I know I could be infertile—but I still get tense about it.'

'I can't understand how women who have irregular periods cope. I only have to be a day late and I can't get it out of my mind.'

'The relief when I felt the usual pains in my stomach was like I used to feel when I passed a test at school.'

'What if I'm pregnant?' There are no figures to show how many women ask themselves that question on any given day, but you don't have to be a statistician to estimate that there are tens of thousands. Unplanned pregnancy is a hazard for every sexually active, fertile woman who does not wish to conceive. And few women have escaped the terror of the 'pregnancy panic', the day when the expected period doesn't start.

We have been trying to control our fertility from the earliest days of civilization, and we still have not succeeded. There is no method of contraception that is one hundred per cent effective—and even if there were it is unlikely that we would always be able to organize our sex lives so as to take advantage of it.

The book has been written for all women at risk of unplanned pregnancy and for all those working with them. It addresses two separate issues: why an unplanned pregnancy happens, and what a woman can do about it when it does.

As a reader, you can use the book in different ways. You may want to read the book from cover to cover or you may just want to dip into particular chapters to extract the information you need.

Chapter 1 contains a discussion of why unplanned pregnancies happen. It shows how an unplanned pregnancy is, in many ways, an accident waiting to happen. Women facing unplanned pregnancies are not stupid, careless, or feckless—they are simply women with a problem. And contrary to popular thinking that problem is typically not of their own making. Some women become unintentionally pregnant despite meticulous use of contraception, others unintentionally expose themselves to risk because they wrongly believe themselves to be using contraceptives effectively.

Often when a woman finds that she is pregnant her first reaction is one of shock and disbelief. One woman, who became pregnant despite using the contraceptive pill, told me that she was stunned because she did not understand how it could have happened; and because she did not understand how she could have conceived, she was scared that it could happen again. By explaining how and why unplanned pregnancies happen, Chapter 1 aims to provide a framework for any woman to understand what could have happened to her.

Chapter 2 discusses the symptoms of pregnancy, and why some women recognize their condition straight away while others remain in ignorance for months.

Chapter 3 looks at the choices that face every woman with an unintended pregnancy and examines why the decision about what to do next is seldom as straightforward as it might seem.

Chapters 4, 5, and 6 examine a woman's options in detail, looking at what is involved in the decisions to have an abortion or to continue with the pregnancy and either keep the child or relinquish it for adoption.

By understanding both our problems and their possible solutions, we can more effectively take control of our lives.

Contents

1

It happens all the time

It is a striking fact that in an age when we can send space shuttles to Mars, build computers smaller than postage stamps' and carry out complex organ transplants, we still can't control our own fertility. Despite modern methods of family planning, and widespread information about how to use it, unplanned pregnancy is one of the most common medical problems faced by sexually active women under 45.

Many tens of thousands of unplanned pregnancies end in abortion, making it the most common operation among women in the fertile age range. Other women decide that, although the pregnancy was accidental, they are able to accommodate a surprise addition to their life. For a small, but significant number of women, the solution to an unplanned pregnancy is to give birth to a child, and allow it to be adopted.

It is impossible to calculate precisely just how many pregnancies each year are accidental. When the medical sociologist, Anne Fleissig, asked a number of women who had given birth six weeks previously whether their pregnancy was planned, she found that 31 per cent of pregnancies were not, and she concluded in a paper subsequently published in the *British Medical Journal*[1] that almost a third of births could be the consequence of accidental pregnancies. If this were the case it would mean 310 000 accidental pregnancies in Britain every year.

This is likely to be a conservative estimate, because Anne Fleissig conducted her research into the circumstances in which women's new babies were conceived, and so her sample did not include women who had conceived but ended the pregnancy by an abortion. These unplanned pregnancies suggest that the real extent of accidental pregnancy is even higher—perhaps as high as 50 per cent of all conceptions.

Defining unplanned pregnancy

It is almost impossible to draw a clear line between those pregnancies that are planned and those that are unplanned.

In the first place, it is difficult to arrange a pregnancy to order. The average fertile couple trying for a child may take three or four months to conceive, and many couples go through a stage where they're not exactly planning to have a child now, but they're not exactly doing everything in their power to prevent it either. Women who use the contraceptive pill are often advised to switch to a barrier method of contraception, such as a diaphragm or condom, three months before they intend to start 'trying' for a child. Barrier methods are inherently less effective and if the couple has difficulty using them, and happens to be highly fertile, it is quite possible that the pregnancy intended for three months hence will arrive sooner than planned. Is this an unplanned pregnancy? Technically, yes.

Then what about the situation where one partner wants a child, but the other is reluctant? A woman may assert her maternal ambitions by frequently 'forgetting' to take her contraceptive pill, thereby becoming pregnant 'accidentally on purpose'. She may always insist that she conceived unintentionally, never admitting that she took chances that she would not have taken had she been committed to avoiding pregnancy. A man can just as easily manipulate things so that risk situations occur. He may 'forget' to buy condoms, insist if they have sex that he will withdraw before ejaculation, and then get 'carried away'; or he may deliberately engineer situations where unprotected sex is likely in some other way. Sometimes these manoeuvres are quite conscious and deliberate, but often they are unconscious and not even recognized by the people who perpetrate them. Are the resulting pregnancies unplanned? Certainly they seem so to one partner, but to the other . . . ?

An 'accidental' pregnancy may even be the consequence of a woman's insecurity about her own fertility. The frequent discussions about infertility in newspapers, women's magazines, and on television may lead some women to doubt their own ability to have a child when the time is right. If a woman who has never had a child frequently reads about the sub-fertility problems of others, and takes to heart the statistic that one couple in six experiences fertility problems, she may well suffer all manner of doubts and fears about her reproductive future. She may not want a child *now* but in the recesses of her subconscious mind she may be desperate to discover if she *can* conceive. She may even develop an irrational belief that she is subfertile and become cavalier as to her contraception as a consequence. This may also lead to an 'accidental' pregnancy.

It is also possible for accidental pregnancies to be disguised as deliberate conceptions. A woman may be embarrassed to admit that a pregnancy is accidental in case she is thought to be stupid, or in case the accident confers some kind of stigma on her future child. Many women feel genuinely ambivalent about their pregnancy and are quite honestly unsure whether it was intended or 'just happened'.

Women face a great many social pressures to have children, and these pressures influence the way we think and feel about our fertility. A woman who confides to a friend that she is pregnant may be so overwhelmed with congratulations—particularly if she is perceived to be in a stable, long-term relationship—that it may be difficult to admit that the pregnancy was neither planned, nor whole-heartedly welcome. To declare, in such circumstances, that her new state is a big mistake may require a degree of boldness beyond what the couple can summon. However, once the pregnancy has been redefined publicly as a 'happy event', it may well become redefined in this way in the minds of the expecting couple.

But in many cases (probably the vast majority of cases) there is no doubt at all about the accidental character of a pregnancy. Women become pregnant in circumstances where they have absolutely no desire to conceive and have done absolutely everything to prevent conception.

A modern risk for all of us

Despite modern contraception, better provision of sex education, and greater scientific knowledge about human reproduction, a number of factors combine to place women today at just as great a risk of unplanned pregnancy as women of our mothers' or grandmothers' generations.

We probably have sex more often, we may have a greater number of partners during our lives, and our expectations of sex are different. Whereas for earlier generations sex was linked to marriage and motherhood, it is now regarded by many in Western society as a legitimate form of recreational, rather than mainly procreational, activity. We do it for fun rather than to 'make babies'. The very notion of unplanned pregnancy rests on the assumption that it is possible to plan pregnancy. Whereas previous generations, having sex without effective modern contraceptives, constantly feared pregnancy, we *expect* to enjoy sex without consequences.

The more times a woman has sex, the greater her chances of falling pregnant. This simple fact means that we may risk accidental pregnancies more than previous generations simply because our active sex life extends over a longer period of time than that of our parents and grandparents. We now start to form sexual relationships at an earlier age and expect to enjoy an active sex life until well beyond the menopause.

Young girls today mature faster, physically and emotionally, and so it is hardly surprising that they explore their sexuality at a younger age. When the sociologist, Michael Schofield, investigated the sexual behaviour of young people in the early 1960s, he found that just two per cent of girls and six per cent of boys claimed to have experienced full sexual intercourse[2]. By 1990, almost a third (31 per cent) of 16 year olds and 70 per cent of 19 year olds were claiming to have had full sexual intercourse[3]. This means that more young women are having sex at a time when their fertility is particularly high, when they may find it difficult to obtain access to family planning services, and have to negotiate the use of contraception with an equally young, inexperienced partner. Young women may feel unable to seek advice about the more effective methods of contraception, such as the pill, because they are worried about their parents finding out—perhaps by discovering a pill packet, or as a consequence of a doctor's breach of confidentiality.

However, it is quite wrong to see unplanned pregnancy as a problem only for young women. Public attention focuses on teenage pregnancies partly because they are ideal subjects for sensational media stories, and partly because they are a particularly vulnerable social group; but older women are also at risk.

It is no longer expected that women in their twenties should be either married and preparing to embark on family life, or on the look-out for a husband. The 20-somethings of the 1990s are likely to be continuing their education, forging careers, or simply enjoying a break between leaving their parents' home and starting their own. Even if a couple settles into a stable heterosexual relationship and achieves a secure income and a decent home, it is still considered normal and appropriate for them to defer having children until their late twenties or early thirties. And all the time that they are deferring a deliberate pregnancy they are at risk of an accidental one.

Whilst previous generations may have assumed that any pregnancy was wanted and deliberate, so long as the couple were married, today's married couples may have other plans which do not include children at all. Society in general still assumes that women will want children at some time in their lives, but an increasing number of couples are deciding that their priorities lie elsewhere and parenthood is not for them.

It is no longer assumed that a married, childless couple are infertile. Recent research suggests that as many as ten per cent of women over the age of 40 are childless through choice, rather than infertility,[4] although, if a couple wish to remain childless and they are fertile, they may face considerable problems, particularly as they may not be able to obtain some of the most effective methods of contraception. Doctors are sometimes reluctant to sterilize couples who have no children, considering that it may be possible that they will change their minds and wish to have a child at some time in the future. And many doctors are loathe to insert IUDs into childless women as the procedure can be more painful than for those who have given birth.

Unplanned pregnancies are not just a problem for those who wish to remain childless. They can be just as great a problem for couples who have planned and had children. Another addition to the family may bring about emotional and financial pressures that are damaging to the couple and their existing children—but a woman struggling to cope with young children may find that organizing her own contraception is the one job that drops from her busy agenda.

Women are at particular risk of accidental pregnancy shortly after the birth of a planned child, when they may be preoccupied with mothering and not yet settled into a new contraceptive regime.

Fertility can return within a few months of childbirth, especially if the new mother is not breastfeeding.

A surprise pregnancy can be a particular nightmare for a woman approaching her menopause. We expect our sex lives to continue until well into old age and, while a woman's fertility level starts to decline from her mid-30s, women can and do get pregnant right up until their menopause. There are many reasons why an unplanned pregnancy at this stage in life can seem disastrous. A couple may resent the thought of having to embark on another round of child-raising just when they were organizing some time for themselves. The woman may be distressed by the knowledge that the child will have a far greater statistical risk of a genetic disability. The couple may worry that they are too old to cope with the stresses and strains of baby-care. Yet as long as they are having sex they are at risk, and that risk may be increased if they have relied on the pill for contraception and the woman has now been advised to change, perhaps because she smokes, to a new, unfamiliar method.

An added difficulty for an older woman with an unexpected pregnancy is that she may mistake the absence of her periods for the start of menopausal symptoms and not identify the problem for months.

Accidental pregnancy is a potential problem for all fertile women who are sexually active. We live in an age in which it is accepted that pregnancies do not just happen by the grace of God or an act of nature. Our lives are organized to incorporate sex for enjoyment and emotional satisfaction, and it is seen as quite normal that we should wish to suppress our fertility. We expect to plan pregnancy just as we expect to be able to plan other aspects of our lives. Unfortunately, keeping our fertility in check is easier to say than to do.

Why accidental pregnancies happen

Contraceptive failure

Contraceptive failure plays a huge part in accidental pregnancy. Anne Fleissig found that over two thirds (69 per cent) of the women in her study who had become unintentionally pregnant claimed to

HQ767.15.B66 2003
    BOONIN, DAVID

HQ767.15.C38 2000
    Cannold, Leslie

HQ1073.P74 2000
    TORR, JAMES

The findings clearly indicate
levels of anxiety and depres
subtypes were compared on
both parents and children us
sizes of approximately 0.5, t
revealed that the effect sizes
ADHD/COM and ADHD/I
negligible to small (less than
of anxiety), ratings for child
children with ADHD/I (mod
significance. Also, when the
of internalizing disorders, th
using dimensional measures
internalizing symptomatolog
not support the contention n
ADHD/I, at least as it is def

Table II. Group Comparisons on N

	ADHD/COM
	M
BASC Anxiety	51.5
BASC Depression (without EXT)	66.7[a]
BASC Depression (with EXT)	61.8
RCMAS (Worry–Oversens.)	10.9[a]
CDI (Neg. mood and Esteem)	49.1

Note. Means and standard deviations are in T score fo
$SD = 3$). Means and standard deviations for BASC De
with EXT as a covariate. Entries for BASC Depression
deviations. Means with varying superscripts differ signi
for multiple post hoc comparisons conducted at $p < 0$.

have been using a method of contraception at the time they conceived. Other research has shown similar results. A study of 769 women requesting abortion in the NHS, conducted by David Bromham, chair of the faculty of Family Planning and Reproductive Health Care of the Royal College of Obstetricians and Gynaecologists found that 68 per cent had conceived as a result of a failure of contraceptive method[5]. A previous study[6] found that of 1 020 women referred for abortions, a fifth claimed to have been using the pill, one of the methods commonly regarded as the most effective.

An authoritative report on unplanned pregnancy by the Royal College of Obstetricians and Gynaecologists[7] acknowledges that contraceptives let couples down, but they also draw attention to the fact that just as contraceptives are fallible, so are we. A contraceptive is only as reliable as the person using it: the most effective contraceptive pill will not prevent pregnancy in the woman who forgets to take it.

The success of a contraceptive method depends on the effectiveness of the method in itself and our ability to use it properly. No method of contraception prevents pregnancy unless it is used in the manner in which the manufacturers intended. It sounds obvious, and in principle it is: in practice things become rather more difficult. This may account for the difference between the very low failure rates for contraceptives quoted by some contraceptive research centres and the manufacturers responsible for their production, and the much higher failure rates that are indicated by some of the studies mentioned above.

There is a world of difference in that way that contraceptives are used in many study conditions—study participants may know that they are part of a trial, are usually highly motivated to use a particular contraceptive, and have been carefully instructed as to what to do—and the circumstances in which most of us actually use contraceptives. This is clearly shown by the different results obtained in two different studies of the effectiveness of methods of contraception.

The most widely quoted study of the failure rates of contraceptives is known as the Oxford Family Planning Study. Published in 1982, it was conducted by Martin Vessey in collaboration with the Family Planning Association[8], and is still regarded as providing the most representative data for the UK.

Vessey calculated the number of women out of 100 who would become pregnant if they used the following methods for a year as being as follows:

Combined pill	0.3
Diaphragm	1.9
Condom	3.6
Spermicide alone	11.9
Periodic abstinence (natural methods)	15.5

However, these results are starkly different from those obtained from a more recent study of contraceptive failure rates in the USA, published in 1992[9].

The authors of this equally reputable study found that the percentage of women who became pregnant within a year, despite having expressed the intention to avoid pregnancy for at least a year, was as follows:

Combined pill	8
Diaphragm	16
Condom	15
Spermicide alone	25
Periodic abstinence (natural methods)	26

How can this vast difference be explained? David Paintin, former editor of the *British Journal of Obstetrics and Gynaecology* and current Chair of the reproductive health information charity, Birth Control Trust, argues that the difference may be explained by the methods used to select the sample of people studied. In a recent paper[10] he explains that the couples studied by Vessey were 'over 25 years old, were in a long-term relationship, were living in better than average socio-economic status and were willing from the late 1960s onwards to return every six months to be interviewed by a research assistant'. Paintin believes that the US study may reflect more accurately the effectiveness of contraceptive methods when used by average couples in normal conditions.

Contraception is not always easy to fit into a normal life-style, and this is particularly true of those methods that are used at the time of sex itself. Positioning a diaphragm in the right place so that it covers the cervix, while easy enough most of the time, can be tricky when you've enjoyed half a bottle of wine and are feeling rushed.

Even methods that can be dealt with in a methodical and routine fashion throw up problems of their own. With a diaphragm or a condom you can at least check to make sure it is in place but if you rely on the contraceptive pill there are no easy checks you can make to ensure it is having the required effect. Even if a woman is sufficiently informed to know that severe stomach upsets may interrupt the pill's action, how is she to judge whether the attack of diarrhoea she had was severe enough to make a difference?

Family planning professionals describe contraceptive failure in two ways: 'method failure' covers incidents when the contraceptive is used according to the letter of the instructions but fails never the less, and 'user failure' covers human error situations, for example forgotten pills, incorrectly applied condoms, or misplaced diaphragms.

Contraceptive failure can be devastating. If a woman has taken a risk and had unprotected sex then she knows there is a possibility that she may be unlucky. However, a contraceptive failure can leave her feeling completely out of control of her life.

A contraceptive failure can leave the couple that experiences it insecure about future sex. If it happened once, then surely it can happen again. If possible, it is important to identify exactly what went wrong. Sometimes there is no apparent explanation, but frequently a reason can be found and locating it restores some degree of control to the couple with the problem pregnancy. At least they can try to avoid repeating the mistake.

Why contraceptives let us down

In the following section the expression 'careful use' implies that the method used is in test conditions, and so reflects the performance of the method in itself. 'Typical use' describes what happens when the method is used taking into account the usual degree of human error. The figures used here are those quoted by the Family Planning Association.

Combined pill

With careful use fewer than one couple in a hundred using this method for a year will become pregnant. With typical use the pregnancy rate can be as high as three couples in a hundred. The possible causes of failure are given below.

Missed pills A recent MORI poll[11] found that 60 per cent of 326 pill users had forgotten to take their pill at least once during the preceding 12 months, while a further seven per cent were unable to say with certainty that they had always remembered.

The combined pill works by suppressing ovulation. If the level of artificial hormones in the body drop below a certain level then the women can become fertile again. Ideally, the pill should be taken at the same time each day, and you can lose contraceptive protection if you take a pill more than 12 hours late.

If you miss one pill, it should be taken as soon as you remember even if it means taking two pills in the same day. If you miss more than one pill, you should take the last missed pill and then take the rest of the packet at the normal time. You need to take extra precautions for seven days. If the seven days run beyond the end of the packet, then a new packet should be started immediately without the usual break.

The most risky pills to miss are those at the beginning and end of the pack.

Stomach upsets Vomiting or severe diarrhoea can interfere with the absorption of the pill and put you at risk of pregnancy. If you suffer from such a problem you should use additional precautions (such as a condom) during the illness and for seven days after.

The pill interacts with other drugs Pregnancy can occur as a consequence of the interaction between the pill and certain other drugs such as some antibacterial and anti-convulsant medications and also, certain analgesics, sedatives, tranquillizers, and antibiotics. Ampicillin, amoxycillin, augmentin, and tetracycline are commonly prescribed antibiotics which may cause problems in some women.

Doctors should always check whether you are on the pill before they prescribe any drug which may react with it, and you should be advised of any precautions you need to take. However, it's not always the case that what *should* happen *does* happen, especially when a doctors is under pressure from a crowded waiting room. It always make sense to remind your doctor that you are taking the pill if she suggests you take another medicine.

Progestogen only pills

With careful use just one couple in a hundred will become pregnant, but with typical use the failure rate rises to four in a hundred.

The possible causes of failure are the following.

You are late taking the pill   You absolutely must take a progestogen only pill at the same time each day. Even a delay as short as three hours could place you at risk of pregnancy. This type of pill suppresses ovulation in fewer than 50 per cent of the women who take it. Instead it works by causing changes in the cervical mucus which make it difficult for the sperm to enter the womb, and making the womb lining less receptive to the egg if it is fertilized. This means that once the level of hormone becomes insufficient to sustain these changes you are immediately put at risk. If a pill is forgotten, it should be taken immediately and the next pill taken when at the usual time, but you need to use additional precautions, as with the combined pill, for seven days.

Maintaining a strict regime to ensure the pill is taken at the correct time can be a nightmare for some women. If you take your pill in the morning there's a chance that you might forget until you get to work. If you take it at night, you may need to remember to take it out with you if a night on the town means you don't know what time you will return. Trips abroad, when you cross time zones, cause all manner of complications.

Stomach upsets   As with the combined pill, vomiting or severe diarrhoea can interfere with the absorption of the progestogen-only pill, and you should use additional precautions during the illness and for the next seven days.

Other drugs block the hormones   Progestogen only pills do not interact with antibiotics. However some other drugs, including some barbiturates, can interfere with the absorption of the hormone.

Weight gain   This is controversial, but there is a possibility that this kind of pill become less effective in women who weigh more than 11 stones (70 kg).

Injections

Contraceptive injections are virtually 100 per cent effective.

Possible reasons for failure are:

Forgetting to return for a repeat injection   A single injection lasts for either 8 weeks or 12 weeks depending on the type of injection used. The doctor will give you a note of the day that you need return for a repeat injection, but if you miss the appointment you may be at risk.

Weight gain   As with the progestogen-only pill it may be the case that this method is less effective for women who weigh more than 11 stone (70 kg).

Many women find that their periods stop altogether or become extremely irregular when they have been using injections for some time. This could mean that if you do become pregnant you may not notice as quickly as with other methods.

Intrauterine Devices (IUDs)

Fewer than two couples in a hundred using an IUD will become pregnant.

Possible reasons for failure include the following.

You don't notice the IUD has been expelled from the womb.   The IUD is a small device made of copper and plastic which is inserted into the womb, leaving a couple of threads coming through the cervix. After your period you need to check these threads to make sure that the IUD has not been expelled with the menstrual blood. This rarely happens, but if it does it leaves you completely unprotected.

Diaphragm

With careful use just one or two couples in a hundred users will have a pregnancy. With typical use as many as 15 couples in a hundred will become pregnant.

Possible reasons for failure include the following.

The diaphragm is incorrectly placed The diaphragm acts as a barrier to prevent sperm from passing through the cervix, so it is vital that the device is placed directly over the cervix. Some women find this very straightforward, but if you find it difficult to feel where your cervix is then placing your diaphragm can be very tricky.

If you gain or lose 7 lbs (3 kg) or more, or if you have an abortion, a miscarriage, or you give birth your diaphragm may no longer fit as exactly as it should, and you will need to be re-examined and maybe 'refitted' by your GP or family planning doctor.

You fail to use spermicide correctly Diaphragms are designed to be used with a spermicide. A little should be spread round the edge and on the side closest to the cervix. You can put the diaphragm in place up to three hours before sex, but more spermicide must be used if a longer period of time elapses or you make love again.

You take the diaphragm out too soon The diaphragm should be left in place for at least six hours after sex (but not longer than 30 hours). If you need to use more spermicide because you intend to have sex again you should use a spermicidal pessary.

The diaphragm is damaged You need to inspect the diaphragm before *every* use for tears or small holes. Oil based products of any kind (including creams to treat infections and massage oils) will damage the diaphragm by breaking down the rubber. Even if no problems are spotted the device should be replaced yearly.

Condoms

With careful use just two couples in a hundred will get pregnant but with typical use as many as 15 couples in a hundred will experience a pregnancy.

The main reasons for failure are:

The condom slips off unnoticed Everybody worries about this but fortunately it does not happen frequently. The man must be quite careful to keep the condom on the penis when he withdraws by holding it firmly at the rim.

The man fails to put it on early enough This is a more common problem. Small amounts of semen can leak from the penis as soon as it is erect, and it needs just one sperm in the wrong place at the wrong time to lead to a pregnancy. The condom must be on before any kind of genital contact whatsoever.

The condom tears or splits Condoms are extremely strong and in the usual course of events very reliable. However, it is easy to snag a condom on fingernails or jewellery when retrieving it from the packet or rolling it on. As with diaphragms, all oil-based products cause condoms to deteriorate very rapidly.

Natural family planning methods

With 'careful use' just two couples out of a hundred will get pregnant, however with typical use the failure rate can lead to as many as 20 pregnancies among a hundred couples.

Possible reasons for failure are:

You fail to abstain or use back up method at the right time Natural family planning methods are based on identifying when ovulation will take place (see p. 40 for a more detailed explanation of this) and avoiding sex at that time. This can be done by measuring the tiny temperature changes that your body undergoes as part of its normal monthly cycle, learning to identify the changes that take place in your cervical mucus as your fertile period approaches, and working out which days are likely to be fertile on the basis of several previous cycles.

Taken together, the combined indications of fertility can be extremely reliable—although each on its own is highly fallible. Temperature changes can be brought about by all kinds of factors, from catching a cold to taking aspirin for a headache. The changes in cervical mucus are slight and easily masked by semen deposits in the vagina. And your cycle can be easily and unexpectedly disrupted by an illness or stress.

Even if the fertile period is correctly identified it may require a super-human act of will to abstain from penetrative sex, especially after a particularly romantic evening or the consumption of a significant quantity of alcohol.

This method also assumes you have a partner who is prepared to defer to your judgement about when to have sex. While this may be an appropriate relationship to have, it would be idealistic to assume that all partnerships could operate in this way.

Having looked at the most common methods of contraception and the reasons why they can fail, it is easier to understand why so many 'accidents' happen.

Myths and misconceptions

Failure to use a contraceptive properly does not imply that either partner is stupid or careless. Doctors often fail to spend the required amount of time carefully instructing people how to use their chosen method most effectively. Embarrassment often prevents people asking the necessary questions. Few people feel completely at ease talking to their doctor about sex, and because we are often reluctant to reveal our own ignorance we avoid raising questions or problems if we think we should know the answer. This leaves us hanging onto a myriad of myths and half-truths about sex and contraception which can put us at risk.

Research by Britain's largest manufacturer of contraceptive pills, Schering Health Care Ltd, shows that women retain all manner of misconceptions about how to take the pill, which are the most dangerous pills to miss, and what to do if a pill is forgotten. Interviewers found that on average a woman on the pill forgets to take it eight times a year. Most of the women questioned knew they had to do *something* when a pill was missed, but very few knew what the something was. Only one pill-user in ten was aware that missing just one pill could place them at risk of pregnancy and fewer than half knew that diarrhoea or stomach upsets could lessen the effectiveness of their contraceptive.

A woman should be able to have her contraceptive queries answered by one of several people. General practitioners and practice nurses, family planning doctors, pharmacists, and help-lines run by organizations like the Family Planning Association and Brook Advisory Centres all have plentiful information available. Most of us, however, find it hard voluntarily to expose our ignorance, and it is easy for a woman busy with the stresses of everyday life to push her concerns out of her mind.

In fact, we are often unaware of the gaps in our knowledge and we hold on to misinformation not realizing it to be false. Fertility is an extremely complex mechanism and it's easy to understand why there are so many confusions about it.

Take these popular myths, for example.

- *You can't get pregnant during your period*

In general it is most unlikely that a woman would become pregnant as a consequence of sex during her period. As chapter 2 explains in some detail, a woman is fertile only around the time at which she ovulates, and if she has a regular 28-day cycle her fertile time is usually mid-way between her periods. However, if a woman has an irregular cycle, or a regular but very short cycle, it is just possible that sperm deposited in her vagina at the time she was bleeding could still be alive to fertilize an egg released shortly afterwards. Consequently if you have unprotected sex at the time of your period you could get pregnant.

- *As you are only fertile for the 24 hours after you ovulate, you need not bother to use a method of contraception for the rest of the month*

It is true that once the egg has been released it must be fertilized within 24 hours if it is to be fertilized at all. But it is not always easy for a woman to know exactly when she ovulates and when she is due to ovulate next. Even women who carefully monitor their own cycle and are aware of the body changes that take place when they release an egg can make mistakes.

- *If you come off the pill it will take you a while to get pregnant because of the build up of hormones*

This is nonsense—as many women who have fallen pregnant after missing just one pill will testify. Today's pills have such a low hormone content that a woman's body returns to its normal level of fertility extremely quickly. Doctors usually advise women to wait for three months after coming off the pill before they conceive but this is simply because it allows the cycle to settle down and so makes it easier for them to date the conception. However, if the woman does not want to conceive immediately she should be advised to use another method of contraception in the intervening period.

Contraceptive manufacturers have tried to improve the 'patient advice' information which is included in pill packets, but such information can only complement a detailed one-to-one discussion with a doctor who has an up-to-date knowledge of contraceptive practice. Leaflets can only deal in generalities and a woman wants to know how her method of contraception is going to affect her as an individual. Many women suffer contraceptive failures because no one has explained to them exactly how to use a method properly.

The importance of clear explanation and motivation in the use of a contraceptive method is shown by the relatively low 'user failure' rate for the progestogen-only pill. This type of pill is considerably more difficult for a woman to use than the more commonly prescribed combined pill. As outlined above, the progestogen-only pill must be taken at the same time each day if it is to be effective—if the user is more than three hours late in taking it she loses protection. Given this it would be reasonable to expect that the user-failure rate would be far higher than the combined pill, but this is not the case. This may partly be because doctors prefer to prescribe progestogen-only pills to older women who may be less fertile, but it may also be the case that prescribers are more aware of the need for progestogen-only pill users to be highly motivated about their pill-taking and so are extra careful to provide such motivation.

Where contraceptives are simply bought from a pharmacist or supermarket there is even less opportunity to discuss exactly how the method should be used. Many people find buying condoms or spermicide excruciatingly embarrassing and would never dream of discussing exactly how they should be used.

Lack of knowledge about contraceptive use is often understood as a problem for young people just discovering sex. There are countless reports identifying the need for better sex education in schools and more support for parents to help to explain the 'facts of life'. Ironically, in some ways, it can be easier for young people to obtain knowledge because once the barrier of bravado has been broken down it is easier for them to admit that they are sexually inexperienced and do not know all the answers. An older woman who has been brought up to believe that 'there are some things one just does not discuss' is unlikely to feel sufficiently confident to discuss with her doctor the side-effects caused by her pills and so may just stop taking them.

It can also be harder for older people to admit to areas of ignorance when they are *expected* to be experts in sex. Where, for example, does a 42-year-old man like James (see box) go for advice about how to use a condom?

It's easy to get it wrong

James—a London based marketing executive

'I'm 42, but I'd never used a condom in my life until last month and I couldn't believe what a performance it was. I thought you just ripped the packet open shoved it on and that was that.

'First I couldn't get the pack open. Then once I'd got it out I tried to fit it over the end of my dick but it wouldn't roll down. After some considerable fumbling. I sussed out it *might* be inside out (I never knew there was an inside out). I tried again, but by the time it was half-way there I was getting so embarrassed I was beginning to lose my erection. It's all very well saying this should be a fun piece of love-play, but to be honest I didn't know the woman I was with all that well, it was the first time I'd strayed in 10 years of marriage, and I was desperately trying to act casual. I ended up pulling it on like a sock. The whole experience was absolutely detestable—the smell of the rubber, the feel of the lubricant was horrible. When I actually got on the job I was completely preoccupied with whether it was going to slip off. It's the only time in my life that I've lost an erection while making love. I was so humiliated I wanted to crawl under the bed.

'I suppose some people wouldn't say that this was a contraceptive failure but believe me it was. The contraceptive failed to let me have sex. Fifteen years ago I'd probably have ridden bareback, if she'd let me, regardless of the consequences. It was only fear of catching something that prevented me from taking the risk this time.'

Annie—33-year-old university lecturer

'When I had my diaphragm fitted the doctor told me to come back and have a new one fitted if it started to look battered, and he carefully showed me how to check it for holes. What he didn't tell me was that I'd need a new fitting if my weight changed.

'As it happens, I'd gained quite a lot of weight five years ago when I went on the pill, and when I came off the pill the pounds fell off again. Maybe this meant the diaphragm never fitted me as it should. Anyway, after I'd been using it for eight months I fell pregnant. I was 10 weeks gone before I knew because my periods had been irregular ever since I came off the pill, and as far as I was concerned I never put myself at risk. In fact I used to use so much spermicide I'm surprised that wasn't enough protection in itself.

'For me, the pregnancy, despite being a shock, wasn't the biggest problem in the world. I'd switched to a diaphragm in the first place because we thought we might want to try for a kid at some time. So it simply brought everything forward. But I have to admit I felt really cheated. It's one thing to get pregnant when you know you've taken a chance, but when you know you've done everything by the book . . . it makes you feel really out of control.'

Failure to use contraception at all

Although much is written about contraceptive failure, modern contraceptives do work well most of the time and a large proportion of unplanned pregnancies probably occur because the couple didn't use a method at all. Medical professionals often estimate that as many as 40 per cent of accidental pregnancies are the consequence of 'non-contraceptive usage'. In a study of more than 1000 women referred for abortion in the mid-1980s, half admitted that they were not using a method of contraception[12].

It may seem difficult to imagine why any woman should put herself at this risk—until you consider the circumstances in which sex takes place. Sex is not always premeditated and often happens in the heat of passion, a consequence of what Britain's only professor of family planning, John Guillebaud, has dubbed the 'moonlight and roses' effect. Suddenly the mood is right and caution is thrown to the wind.

Sex is still surrounded by stigma and taboos. Even in these post-Madonna times men are supposed to be the 'seducers' and women the 'seduced'. Sex is supposed to take place as a spontaneous act of love and emotion and being prepared, with a packet of condoms in your handbag, reveals that you had anticipated it. The possibility of sex is something that neither partner may wish to admit, especially if the relationship is in its early stages, or one or both partners feel uncomfortable about sex in general or their sexuality in particular. It is often suggested that people who are emotionally uncomfortable about sex are more likely to have unplanned pregnancies because they are less likely to possess accurate information about conception and contraception. They are also less likely to acknowledge that they may have sex in the near future, less likely to take steps to obtain contraception, less likely to communicate about sex with their partner, and less likely to use a chosen method of contraception consistently.

However, there must be thousands of women who are quite comfortable with their sexuality, but have found themselves unable to use contraception even though they knew they were taking a chance. Sometimes, no matter how organized we are, as Frances and Jackie discovered (see box), life throws up the unexpected.

Frances—22-year-old personnel secretary

'I was always pretty paranoid about getting pregnant and started on the pill even before I started to have sex. I knew I'd sleep with a boy sooner or later, so it made sense to be prepared for it. I only ever took a chance once.

'Gary and I had a huge row. I found out that he had been seeing someone else and that was it as far as I was concerned—the end. We'd been living together but I told him to get out and he did. I was really upset, but I couldn't put up with that sort of dishonest behaviour. It seemed really sordid. I stayed on the pill, out of habit more than anything else. You get used to taking them without really thinking about it.

'I usually went to the clinic for a repeat prescription at the start of my last pack, but as it happened I was away that week, then I was too busy to get time off work and then . . . there didn't really seem any point anyway. I hadn't got a boyfriend any more and I wasn't interested in anyone. It seemed a bit unnecessary to be taking all those hormones when I didn't need them. When I'd started on the pill the first time it seemed as though it was 'the thing to do,' all my friends were doing it 'just in case', but I guess when you get older you don't think about sex and boys all the time and it's easier to put it to the back of your mind.

'Anyway, I'd been off the pill for about six weeks when I came back from the cinema to find Gary waiting in the car outside the flat. I guess we just looked at each other and that was that. It was the most romantic thing that had ever happened to me. He swore he'd made the biggest mistake of his life and that he really loved me. I definitely still loved him. Of course we ended up making love. I never even thought about the consequences—I'd never had to before. It never occurred to him that I'd come off the pill.

'As it happens we were lucky. Nothing happened as a result, but the rest of the month was murder. I was so relieved when my period started.'

Jackie—34-year-old social worker

'Even at the time we made love I knew I was taking a huge gamble, but even though it sounds really corny, I have to say I couldn't help myself.

'I had gone away with a colleague to a conference. I had fancied him for ages but I didn't think for a minute we would sleep together because I knew he was married and really happy with his wife and kids. At home I used condoms with my boyfriend, I used to buy them and often carried them around with me—but not on this trip. It didn't even cross my mind.

'Anyway there was a lot of drinking and laughing and some of us went to a nearby club. John and I stayed on when everyone else left but even when we left to go back to the hotel together I don't think it was clear to either of us that we would have sex. We hadn't even kissed, we had just danced together. He kissed me for the first time in the lift and one thing, as they say, led to another. I think he assumed I was on the pill or something, and although I knew I was being stupid I couldn't bear to say 'stop', and insist he found a condom. I knew if we stopped that would be it—he would get all guilty and I'd have to go back to acting like the responsible professional woman I have to be most of the time.

'It was just a one night stand and when I found I was pregnant I was wrecked. I never told a soul not even John.'

Barrier methods of contraception are a minefield of modern etiquette problems. At exactly what stage of sex play do you mention that you have to insert your diaphragm or you want him to wear a condom? Who is expected to carry the condoms? If you are going on holiday alone is it sensible to pack your diaphragm or a packet of condoms?

The answers are, of course, available in all manner of leaflets, booklets, and magazine articles. We are instructed to make our contraceptive and prophylactic intentions known as soon as 'intimate relations' become a possibility, women are to be seen as sensible rather than sluts if they prepare for sex and take the contraceptive initiative. But life is generally not so clear cut, and endless surveys show that even though a growing number of people carry condoms they often remain unused in the packet. Just because we know we *should* use contraception doesn't mean we actually do.

Contraceptive availability

Even if their intentions are good, a couple may not be able to take contraceptive action if they cannot obtain their favoured contraceptive when they need to use it. Access to contraceptive advice and supplies remains a problem for many couples.

Condoms are the most easily available one of the various methods. Over the last ten years it has become much easier to obtain them. Not only are they sold in chemists and supermarkets but a growing number of machines are appearing in public toilets and in pubs, bars, clubs, colleges, and even some enlightened work-places. However, we are still some way away from the openness demonstrated in France where condom machines are to be found on busy streets.

Contraceptives methods which are only available on prescription can pose more of a problem for women. Even the most conscientious pill-user is likely to have experienced that moment of panic when she realizes that she has lost or used up the spare packet of pills that she could have sworn was safely tucked away in the bathroom cabinet.

In principle it should be easy to obtain a prescription for the pill, or to have a diaphragm or an IUD fitted, as almost all GPs provide a family planning service and there is a widespread network of family planning clinics. In practice it can be more difficult. Many family planning clinics are open for fewer than two sessions a week, often at times that are extremely inconvenient for the women who wish to use them. A clinic that is open between 2 pm and 4 pm on a Thursday afternoon is of little use to a working woman who is unable to pop out for a couple of hours. A recent survey conducted by Brook Advisory Centres[13] found that 44 per cent of teenagers requesting contraceptive help from family planning clinics were unable to get an appointment within a week.

Young people have a particular need for an alternative source of contraceptives to their GP—especially in smaller towns and villages where the GP may know their family well. GPs are, of course, bound by strict regulations concerning confidentiality, but a teenager trying to obtain the contraceptive pill without her parents knowledge may be terrified that even if the GP doesn't spill the beans, she may run in to Auntie Maud or her next-door neighbour in the waiting room.

Over the last couple of years many health authorities have decided to orient family planning clinic sessions towards younger women in response to the massive amounts of publicity about teenage pregnancies. While this may have improved services for teenagers, it has sometimes been at the expense of running a decent service for older women, as general clinics have been cut to allow special 'young persons' clinics to be set up.

Cost-cutting within the National Health Service can also mean that it is more difficult to get your chosen contraceptive method without paying for the 'privilege'. A whole range of services are affected. It is become increasingly difficult to be sterilized without having to pay to have the operation privately. In some areas couples can expect to wait up to 18 months for a vasectomy operation, in others it is not available on the NHS at all and the waiting lists for female sterilization operations is even longer. GPs and family planning clinics are under growing pressure to prescribe the cheapest brands of contraceptive pill, despite the fact that they might be less-well tolerated by the woman for whom they are prescribed. The fewer problems a contraceptive method causes a woman, the more likely she is to use it effectively, and this particularly applies to the pill. The greater the number of side-effects suffered by a woman the less motivated she will be to take it regularly. Over the last few years new formulations of hormones have been created which lessen the risk of the side-effects like weight gain, headaches, and breakthrough bleeding, that affected some women. Unfortunately these newer, better pills are more expensive and because of the financial pressure on whom? Doctors? GPs? There are suggestions that many are avoiding these newer brands.

Post-coital contraception

Greater availability of emergency post-coital contraception could significantly dent the numbers of accidental pregnancies by providing a second chance for women who know they are at risk. There are two ways of preventing pregnancy after sex has taken place. One involves the insertion of an IUD within five days of sex, which can be removed when the woman has her next period. The more common method involves two doses of a special pill. The two doses are taken 12 hours apart, but the first must be within 72 hours of sex.

The emergency contraceptive pill is available from most doctors and family planning clinics and from some Accident and Emergency departments of local hospitals. It is however significantly under-utilized because of the misconceptions that surround the way it should be used. For example, many women assume that if they have been advised by a doctor that they cannot take the normal contraceptive pill they will be unable to use the emergency pill. This is not the case, as most problems caused by the normal pill are a consequence of taking the hormone over a long period of time, whereas this pill involves a short higher dose. Unfortunately media coverage of emergency contraception often refers to it as the 'morning after pill' which fuels another misconception—that it must be taken the morning after sex. Consequently many women who could take advantage of it believe they have missed their chance.

Even given the 72 hours in which emergency contraceptive pills can be used, you may find it difficult to obtain an appointment with a doctor who can issue the tablets. Most women have had the experience of telephoning their GP for an emergency appointment only to be told that earliest available appointment is in four days' time. Under pressure, when it is made clear that there really is an emergency it is usually possible to get a same-day appointment. But this requires a persistence and determination that many women do not have. Not all acts of unprotected sex lead to a pregnancy and so emergency contraception is a safeguard against something that might not happen any way. Many women, faced with difficulties in obtaining it, give up and trust to chance.

Contraception in the real world

Each difficulty a woman has in obtaining effective contraception increases her risk of unplanned pregnancy. Few couples will be prepared to postpone having sex for a week while they wait for an appointment at a clinic. If a woman's brand of contraceptive pill causes her discomfort she is less likely to continue taking it and may switch to a less reliable method of contraception. If a young woman feels a visit to a family doctor for a pill prescription is likely to betray the fact that she is having sex to people from whom she would prefer to keep the fact a secret, she is less likely to make that visit.

In the final analysis contraception is something we all employ reluctantly. We don't take the pill, use a condom, or have an IUD fitted because we want to engage in that activity in its own right but as a precaution—to allow us to enjoy sex without pregnancy. We weigh up the pros and cons—the hassle of using a contraceptive appropriately is balanced against the fear of becoming pregnant. Any disincentives to use a method, whether it be the problem of obtaining it or unhappiness with the way a method makes us feel, all help tip the balance against effective contraceptive usage.

Women who have accidental pregnancies are not stupid, they are not necessarily careless, and are certainly not feckless or irresponsible. Unplanned pregnancy is a potential hazard for every fertile, sexually active woman. The only way to remain 100 per cent safe from the threat of unplanned pregnancy is to restrict sex to those times when you want to conceive: a choice of life-style that most of us would find unacceptable.

The risk of unplanned pregnancy hangs over most of us, and at some time in our lives many of us will run out of luck and face the anguish of a pregnancy test that confirms our worst fears. No amount of regrets, remorse, or self-reproach will change the chemical reaction in a positive test. You can't relive the last month, but you can take control of the future. The choices you make now will affect your life for ever.

References

1. Fleissig, A. (1991). Unintended pregnancy and the use of contraception: changes from 1984 to 1989. *British Medical Journal*, **302**, 147.
2. Michael Schofield (1965). *The sexual behaviour of young people*. Penguin, Harmondsworth.
3. Health Education Authority/Mori (1991). *Adults' health and lifestyles—sexual health*. Health Education Authority, to be published (cited in Report of the RCOG working party on unplanned pregnancy, Royal College of Obstetricians and Gynaecologists).
4. Johnson, G. (1993). Childless women revisited. *British Medical Journal*, **307**, 1116–17.
5. Bromham, D.R. and Cartmill, R.S.V. (1993). Are current sources of contraceptive advice adequate to meet changes in contraceptive practice? A study of patients requesting termination of pregnancy. *British Journal of Family Planning*, **19**, 179–83.
6. Wheble, A.M., Street, P., and Wheble, S.M. (1987). Contraception: failure in practice. *British Journal of Family Planning*, **13**, 40–45.
7. Report of the RCOG Working Party on Unplanned Pregnancy (1991), p. 42. Royal College of Obstetricians and Gynaecologists, London.
8. Vessey, M., Lawless, M., and Yeats, D. (1982). Efficacy of different contraceptive methods. *Lancet*, **8276**, 841–43.
9. Jones, E.F. and Forrest, J.D. (1992). Contraceptive failure rates based on the 1988 National Survey of Family Growth. *Family Planning Perspectives*, **24**, 12–19.
10. Paintin, D. (1994). Why abortion services are necessary. In: D. Paintin (ed.) *Abortion services in England and Wales: How to meet the needs of women and the health service*, pp. 17–18. BCT, London.
11. MORI Consumer Survey of 1258 women aged 16 to 49, throughout the UK, conducted in March and April 1993 on behalf of Roussel Laboratories Ltd.
12. Wheble, A.M., Street, P., and Wheble, S.M. (1987). Contraception: failure in practice. *British Journal of Family Planning*, **13**, 40–5.
13. Brook Advisory Centres (1991). *Annual Report*.

2

Discovering you are pregnant

There are women who claim to have known that they were pregnant even before they missed their first period. Some even insist that they knew immediately they conceived, while some books on pregnancy adopt the tone that although there may be many times in your life when you think might be pregnant, you will *know beyond doubt* when you are.

In reality most women are usually not that certain. Even when a woman has had a wanted pregnancy confirmed by a home test or her doctor, it is common for her to go through weeks of self-doubt about whether she really is pregnant, or is still pregnant. Often it is not until a woman has seen her fetus on a scan or felt it move inside her that she can accept without question that she is going to have a child.

Most women *do* experience some clinical symptoms early in pregnancy, but without the confirmation of a pregnancy test or an examination by an experienced doctor it is difficult to be sure about their cause. Every woman experiences the symptoms of early pregnancy differently, and a further complicating factor is, that many of the most common signs—swollen, tender breasts, tiredness, bloatedness, and weepiness—are extremely similar to the pre-menstrual symptoms that many women suffer every month. Many women spend the early weeks of pregnancy convinced that their period is about to start at any moment.

When we read the occasional reports, in womens' magazines, of women who do not realize that they are pregnant until a very late stage, we often wonder how a woman could possibly remain ignorant of such dramatic changes in her own body. In reality, especially if a woman does not think she could be pregnant, or she is reluctant to face up to the fact, it is possible to mistakenly attribute the symptoms of pregnancy to another cause altogether. Even some of the very obvious signs of pregnancy, such as weight gain and the 'pregnant shape' can be explained away in other ways. Some women's weight gain in pregnancy is slight, and many women who have trouble keeping their weight down may be genuinely convinced that a weight increase of 22 to 28 lbs (the amount most women would expect their weight to increase by while pregnant) is a consequence of losing control over calories rather than having lost control over fertility. Very occasionally, even a slim woman can carry a pregnancy to term without a noticeable change in shape if her uterus lies at an unusual angle, and most obstetricians seem able to remember at least one case of a woman whose initial labour pains were mistaken for a hernia, appendicitis, or indigestion. There are even reports of a midwife whose surprise pregnancy was discovered when she was rushed into casualty at the Chelsea and Westminster Hospital in London with abdominal pains which turned out to be labour pains.

If you have any reason to believe that you could be pregnant and you have any of the symptoms described below it is important to confirm whether or not you are pregnant. This is particulary true if you continue to feel pre-menstrual for longer than usual, but your period doesn't come or is lighter than usual, and the pre-menstrual feeling continues even after your bleed.

Symptoms of early pregnancy: what to look for

In early pregnancy most women experience a combination of some of the following symptoms. While some women suffer from all of them, others do not notice any changes in the first few months.

Missed period

For most women a missed menstrual period will be a sure sign that she is pregnant and often a missed period will draw attention to other symptoms of early pregnancy (see below) which she may have pushed to the back of her mind, or not noticed at all. But although pregnancy is the most common cause of amenorrhoea (absence of periods) in women aged between 15 and 40, there are other reasons why a woman's periods can be delayed or stop altogether and unless she is worried that she may have been at risk of pregnancy, alternative explanations may seem more probable.

Many women suffer irregular bleeding for a variety of reasons, from hormone imbalances to uterine problems such as polyps. For some women this is just the way their body works. It is usual for women to experience irregular periods at the beginning, and towards the end, of their fertile lives, and this may make a missed period due to pregnancy particularly difficult to identify. If a woman approaching her menopause misses a period she may simply put it down to her time of life, and a young girl may not even notice a missed period if her cycle is usually erratic.

It is also usual for women using progestogen-based methods of contraception to have an irregular bleeding pattern. Most women relying on injections of Depo Provera will find that their periods cease after about a year of use, as will a third of women taking the progestogen-only pill. Women using contraceptive implants usually find that they bleed more, rather than less, frequently. But even with this method some women find they bleed very infrequently if at all. It is possible for women who don't notice a missed period to progress quite far into a pregnancy without it even crossing their minds that they are expecting.

If a woman knows that her bleeding pattern is likely to be disturbed by a contraceptive, she will probably be even less concerned by a delayed bleed than a woman who simply has an irregular cycle, and a woman who always has a naturally irregular cycle is unlikely to be as concerned as a woman who can time her periods to the hour. After all, contraception is supposed to be reliable, and she is confident that she has used her chosen method correctly she is unlikely to suspect that she is pregnant.

To further complicate matters, a period-like bleed is not a guarantee that a woman is *not* pregnant. It is estimated that some half of all pregnant women experience a bleed at some time during pregnancy and approximately one-third of pregnant women experience a slight bleed at the time when the developing embryo implants into the lining of the womb. Implantation usually takes place between 10 and 14 days after fertilization, just at the time that a woman would expect her period if she has a cycle of around 28 days. This 'implantation bleed' can easily be mistaken for menstruation especially if the woman usually has light periods.

Tender, swollen breasts

Many women find that swollen, tender breasts are the first obvious sign that they have conceived. This change is usually caused by the increase in the amount of the hormone progesterone, and is particularly likely if a woman's breasts usually swell during the latter half of her menstrual cycle. Often the nipples may tingle, or feel sore, this can also be a response to altered hormone levels and to the increased blood flow to the breasts.

However, it may be difficult for a woman to recognize this as an early sign of pregnancy if she regularly suffers from swollen or sore breasts as a pre-menstrual symptom.

Tiredness

This is often identified as a sign of pregnancy only in retrospect, by a woman who at the time had wondered why she found it so difficult to get up in the morning and keep her eyes open at night. This tiredness (known by doctors as narcolepsy) is thought to be due to the increased production of progesterone which has a slight sedative effect. The tiredness may be a natural defence mechanism, causing the body to slow down and conserve energy to nurture the developing embryo.

Nausea and/or vomiting

This usually starts about four weeks into the pregnancy (two weeks after the first missed period) and lasts for six to eight weeks. Morning sickness, as it is commonly called, can occur at any time during the day, but it is usually made worse by rapid movements (such as getting out of bed) or by having an empty stomach. Nausea can also be accompanied by excessive salivation (hyperptylism).

About two thirds of pregnant women suffer from these symptoms to a greater or lesser degree. Some women suffer so badly that they risk dehydration and need to be hospitalized. The true cause of morning sickness is not fully understood although many doctors think it could be a response to the rising levels of pregnancy hormones, especially human chorionic gonadotrophin (hCG). Others think nausea is a psychosomatic response to pregnancy. If hCG is responsible, it would explain why it does not usually persist after the first three months of pregnancy, when the production of hCG begins to decline.

Increases in vaginal fluids

Many women find that their vaginal fluids become more copious than normal in response to their raised hormone levels. Some find they start to have a brownish, or pinkish tinged vaginal discharge. This is caused by slight changes to the cells on the cervix (neck of the womb), known as a cervical erosion. This is quite harmless and often occurs in non-pregnant women, especially those who take a combined contraceptive pill.

Weepiness

Many women feel very emotional and weepy in the early weeks— whether the pregnancy was planned or not, wanted or unwanted. This may be an effect of the pregnancy hormones, or it may be because any newly pregnant woman is under a great deal of pressure and may feel very under-confident about how she will bear up to the future—whether she intends to continue or to end the pregnancy.

Needing to urinate more often

As early as one week after conception a pregnant woman may feel that she has to empty her bladder more often than usual. Again, this is a consequence of the surging pregnancy hormones. Later in pregnancy the frequent need to pass water is caused by pressure on the bladder from the growing fetus.

Changes in appetite

Some women find that they are ravenous throughout the first weeks of pregnancy. It is common for women to 'go off' certain foods, particularly alcohol, and crave others. Many women notice a metallic taste in their mouths.

There are many theories about food cravings in pregnancy. Some experts maintain that it is a subconscious, psychological response of the pregnant woman, reflecting her need to put herself at the centre of attention—perhaps by making demands on her partner to obtain special foods at inconvenient times. Others agree that the cravings have a psychological character but believe they are triggered by the woman's need for signs to reaffirm the 'fact' of her pregnancy before she is able to detect fetal movement. Other theories suggest that there is a physiological trigger for the food cravings, and that it may be that a woman craves things which she instinctively knows are high in vitamins or minerals in which she may be deficient. This is thought to provide a rationale for why some women crave the chance to munch on non-foodstuffs such as lumps of coal.

Changes in weight

Despite the fact that the embryo is still tiny, some women find they gain an unusual amount of weight in early pregnancy. This may be because a pregnant woman's metabolism slows down with the result that she burns less energy and is more inclined to convert her calorie intake to fat. Or it may simply be that she eats more.

Some women are surprised to find that they actually lose weight in early pregnancy, often because nausea makes it difficult to enjoy food.

It is normal to experience all the above symptoms of early pregnancy, but it is just as normal not to experience any of them.

In *Pregnancy and Childbirth*[1], her bible for mothers-to-be, Sheila Kitzinger observes that many of the symptoms of early pregnancy are culturally specific: in other words women from different cultures have different signs that they are pregnant. In the UK, morning sickness is the sign most expected, while in many under-developed countries women 'know' they are pregnant when they begin to suffer from boils. This may be because our different ways of living expose women to different risks. So a weakened immune system, a natural by-product of pregnancy, may have little effect on women in the UK, where nearly all women can enjoy a nutritious diet, sanitary living conditions, and clean water, but may predispose women living in less developed surroundings to just such conditions as boils.

However, there may also be a psychosomatic component to some of the early pregnancy symptoms. It seems to be the case that when society expects individuals with a certain condition to act in a particular way, they are more likely to fulfil these expectations. This is certainly true of pregnancy, where many women are more likely to suffer symptoms when they have had a pregnancy confirmed. Of course this may be because once the pregnancy has been confirmed, the physical sensations which they have tried to shrug off, are then legitimized and seen as normal.

Everyone's experience of early pregnancy is different

'I honestly did not notice a thing. My period didn't come but other than that there was nothing to tell me that I was expecting.'

'I was sure that my period was due to start any day because I felt so pre-menstrual. I had all the symptoms I usually get before my period, only more-so.'

'I was a bit taken back because my periods are usually as regular as clockwork and I usually get quite bad cramps for a few hours before I bleed. This time, not only did my period start earlier but there were no cramps at all. Not only that, but I usually come on very heavy at first, and this time it was light—more like the last day. After a couple of days the period seemed to stop and I didn't think about it until I noticed that my bra was really tight. When I did a pregnancy test it was definitely positive.'

'I just felt so tired and run down. When my period didn't start I wondered if it was because I had been overdoing it. Things had been really bad at work and I read somewhere that stress can mess up your periods.'

'I didn't notice anything until my period was late, but my husband did. He said that there was definitely something different about me, but he couldn't work out what it was.'

'I kept waiting to be sick or something, but there were none of the signs you hear about, at all. If it hadn't been for that fact that my period didn't come I'd never have known I was expecting until the first scan. I did four home pregnancy tests in the second month because it didn't seem possible.'

'I've had three babies, and each time I first knew I was pregnant when my bra didn't fit. My bosom seems to inflate overnight.'

Women who are absolutely confident that they cannot possibly be pregnant, perhaps because they have been sterilized or because they believe themselves to be infertile, may be the least likely to recognize

the symptoms of early pregnancy—simply because they are not looking for them. In hind-sight they will often realize that they felt
slightly peculiar but at the time they would have attributed it to
something else.

Taking the test

A pregnancy test is the most reliable way to confirm a pregnancy.
Most work by testing for the presence of a pregnancy hormone,
human chorionic gonadotrophin (hCG), in a sample of urine. This
hormone is produced by the body shortly after the pregnancy is
established. Its concentration in the urine rises rapidly in early pregnancy, from around 100 units per millilitre on the first day of a
missed period to a peak of more than 160 000 units per millilitre at
the end of the first three months. It can also be detected in a pregnant
woman's blood.

The hCG hormone stimulates the production of hormones essential for the sustenance of the fetus in early pregnancy. After the sixteenth week the levels of hCG begin to fall and other hormones take
over the regulation of the pregnancy.

Today's pregnancy tests are sufficiently sensitive to detect the presence of hCG in a pregnant woman's urine from the first day of a
missed period until the sixteenth week of pregnancy and are around
99 per cent accurate.

The technology which allows modern pregnancy tests to be so sensitive, fast, and accurate is relatively new, and has only been made
widely available in home test kits in the last decade or so. Before
then, pregnancy tests involved complicated procedures in hospital
laboratories. Until the 1960s, the most common test involved inject-
ing the woman's urine into a rabbit or a toad, and then waiting to
inspect its ovaries. This was costly, time-consuming, and inconvenient for the woman who was often kept waiting for days for the
result. The next generation of tests depended on observing certain
reactions when a small amount of the urine sample was mixed with
certain chemicals. This was observed either on a glass slide under a
microscope or in a test tube. This was much more convenient than
handling toads, but these tests were only able to identify relatively

high levels of hCG, and required the woman to wait for two weeks from the day her period was due, for a result which was just 90 per cent accurate.

Most of the tests used today used sophisticated monoclonal antibody technology. Highly specific antibodies to hCG are used to trigger a signal such as a colour change, if it is present.

Pregnancy tests are available from pharmacies, GPs, family planning clinics, women's health clinics, and commercial pregnancy testing services.

Home tests

Home pregnancy tests are easily available from chemists and are extremely simple to use.

Some involve the collection of a sample of your urine which you then mix with a reagent according to the instructions supplied with the kit. You then place a special plastic indicator in the urine sample for a variable amount of time, depending on how many days late your period is. If you are pregnant, the tip of the indicator changes colour.

The more modern tests work by using a dip-stick which you either hold into the stream of urine, or dip it in a sample of urine which you have collected. The urine is then drawn up the stick over a chemical strip which changes colour if hCG is present. The result can be seen in around five minutes and is usually quite clear. *Any* sign of a colour change, however slight, is a positive result. You may only have traces of hCG in your blood, but you can't have 'traces' of pregnancy—you are either pregnant or you are not.

If you are conducting a test within a week of your period being due, you should use an early-morning sample of urine (the first you pass of the day) as the hormone levels are more concentrated. If, for some reason this is not possible, always test with urine that has been in your bladder for at least four hours.

Home tests are expensive, costing between £8 and £11, but for many women this is a small price to pay for the immediate results and the privacy that they offer. The 'dip-stick' tests are so easy and convenient to use that it is possible to perform a pregnancy test anywhere where there are toilet facilities—at work, in a public convenience, even on a train! This may be important if you are trying to conceal the fact that you may be pregnant from those you live with.

However, while privacy can be an advantage for some women, it can be a disadvantage for others and it may be a drawback not to have professional advice immediately available. Some pregnancy counsellors advise women carrying out home tests to have a partner or friend at hand to share the good or bad news.

GPs and family planning clinics

In theory it is possible to have a free pregnancy test carried out by a GP or at a family planning clinic—but what is possible in theory is not always possible in practice.

Some GPs are reluctant to perform pregnancy tests because they feel that limited NHS resources could be better spent on other things, and that doctors should rely on their skills in examining women. Even without the evidence of a positive pregnancy test, a doctor should be able to confirm a pregnancy by an internal examination, to detect changes in the position of the cervix and the size and position of the uterus at about four weeks gestation (or two weeks after a missed period).

A recent survey of 60 general practices[2] found that just 37 per cent offered a pregnancy testing service and it was not revealed how many of these were free or, if payment was required, what fee was charged. Even when GPs do provide free pregnancy testing they sometimes use older-style tests which are cheaper but less sensitive and may not be accurate until your period is at least 14 days late. If your GP has to send your sample to a hospital laboratory it may be a further two weeks before the result is available.

Some GPs, however, run an exceptionally good service, using the modern home-style tests and can provide an immediate result. Family planning clinics also usually provide an immediate and free service but some restrict it to women who are already registered with them for contraceptive services. Brook Advisory Centres offer free tests to young women. These services have the advantage that practical help and advice is immediately available whatever the result.

Pharmacies and commercial services

Pharmacies sometimes do their own pregnancy testing services. Those which do usually display a notice advertising the fact in their window. The cost and the result time varies.

Commercial pregnancy testing services are to be found in many larger cities and are usually listed in the telephone directory under 'pregnancy testing'.

Not-for-profit clinics

British Pregnancy Advisory Service (BPAS), Pregnancy Advisory Service (PAS), and Marie Stopes Clinics all offer immediate pregnancy testing for less than the cost of a home test. They also offer specialist counselling, help, and advice, whatever the result, if required.

Agencies which oppose abortion

'Life' and some other agencies which oppose abortion sometimes offer free pregnancy testing and advice, but they will not help you to arrange an abortion. However, if you are certain that, should you find yourself pregnant, you would not wish to consider an abortion they may be a useful source of help.

The confirmation that a woman is pregnant can come as a tremendous shock, even if she strongly suspected her condition

---

If you go to any of the above centres you should be prepared to provide the date of your last period and the details of any drugs you are taking—including your method of contraception.

Your method of contraception will not interfere with the accuracy of the result, but knowing what you usually use will alert a doctor to a particular issue he or she may need to discuss. Tell your doctor if you have used a method of emergency 'after sex' contraception (sometimes called the morning-after pill) to try to prevent the pregnancy. There is, however, no evidence to suggest that when emergency contraceptive pills fail they cause damage to the fetus.

beforehand. A positive pregnancy test translates a strong suspicion into a hard fact. Whether the pregnancy is wanted or unwanted, when the test kit changes colour everything changes with it. The hoping and wishing are over—now there are hard practicalities to deal with. Most women feel a strong sense of shock often tinged with disbelief.

Even a negative pregnancy test can trigger a strong emotional response. Feelings of relief can be tinged with feelings of regret and self-doubt, especially when the woman had been pretty certain that she was pregnant or there was no other apparent reason for the delayed period. A negative pregnancy test may provoke all kinds of other worries including, sometimes, irrational fears about whether it is possible for her to get pregnant when she wants to. Having lived with the fact that she *may* be pregnant the confirmation that it is, after all, a false alarm may seem to be an anti-climax.

False negative results from pregnancy tests are rare. Sometimes the test may appear negative if a woman's hormone levels are very low or her urine is particularly dilute when she conducts it. In these circumstances it may take longer for a colour change to show up on the test and it may help to inspect it again after 30 minutes or so. If the test still *looks* negative at this stage it probably *is*. However, if the overdue period has not arrived within three or four days it is sensible to repeat the test. Some home testing packs provide two tests to allow for this.

False positive results almost never happen and it is safe to assume that if there is a colour change in a home test, or you receive a positive result from someone who has conducted a test for you then you are pregnant.

Sometimes, however, a positive test result is obtained in the very early days after a missed period but is then followed by what seems like a delayed period. This may be a sign that a very early miscarriage has taken place. If this happens, it does not indicate that you are prone to future miscarriages or will be unable to conceive in the future, and it usually requires no medical treatment—had the pregnancy test not been taken, this would probably be explained away as a 'late period', rather than a suspected pregnancy.

Miscarriages in very early pregnancy are extremely common. Most doctors estimate that as many as one pregnancy in every four or five end this way, often before the pregnancy has been confirmed. In most cases, these very early miscarriages are probably the body's way of dealing with defective embryos. Pregnancies that have been detected by an hCG test, but that fail to develop to the point where they can be detected by a doctor conducting a physical examination or on a scan are sometimes referred to as 'chemical pregnancies'.

The pregnant body: a biology lesson

It is hardly surprising that some women 'feel pregnant' very soon after conception given the changes that take place in the body. The changes detected by pregnancy tests or by a doctor during an examination are only a small part of the physical transformation taking place.

To understand what happens during early pregnancy it is helpful to roll the clock back and start at the beginning of the monthly reproductive cycle, because it is at this stage that the body is 'set up' for pregnancy. If an egg is not released in that cycle, or it fails to fertilize, the body disengages the pregnancy-alert.

We often think of three 'key events' in early pregnancy: the release of an egg, its fertilization, and the implantation of the early embryo into the lining of the womb. However, these specific stages can only take place if other conditions are right. Preparation for a potential pregnancy actually begins on the first day of a woman's monthly cycle: the day her period starts.

Preparation for pregnancy

It is useful to look at the changes that prepare a woman's body for pregnancy in the following stages:

(1) the days before ovulation;
(2) the fertile period—the days around ovulation;
(3) the post-ovulatory stage.

(1) The days before ovulation

The path to pregnancy starts in the brain. On the first day of menstruation the hypothalamus (the part of the brain that controls basic bodily functions like hunger and thirst) releases a special hormone known as LH–RH (luteinising hormone–releasing hormone). Hormones are the body's chemical messengers. They circulate in the blood and trigger responses. LH–RH prompts the pituitary gland, which is situated at the base of the brain, to produce another hormone known as follicle stimulating hormone (FSH). FSH then seeps into the blood stream and is carried to the ovaries where it gives the signal for hundreds of follicles (small balls of cells with an unripe egg in the middle) to start to grow and ripen.

One follicle always responds to the FSH better than the others and surges ahead. When this happens the other follicles die back. As the single follicle ripens it produces large amounts of the hormone oestrogen which is absorbed into the blood stream. The oestrogen stimulates the cervix, the passage between the vagina and the womb, to start producing wet, stretchy, sperm-friendly mucus. For many women, the change in their vaginal secretions from being thick and sticky (like wall-paper paste) to wet and stretchy (like raw egg white), is the main sign that an egg is being prepared for release. Oestrogen also triggers changes in the endometrium (lining of the womb) causing it to thicken.

(2) The fertile period

The oestrogen produced by the follicle is carried in the blood to the brain where it tells the pituitary gland to stop producing FSH and start churning out another hormone called luteinising hormone (LH). The LH seeps into the bloodstream where it is transported to the ovaries. The follicle containing the egg is now bulging from the surface of one of the ovaries, and at this stage it is usually about the size of a pea. When it feels the LH around it, the follicle ruptures and releases the egg. This 'egg release' is what is known as ovulation. In the day before ovulation, one woman in ten usually experiences tenderness around the ovary and, sometimes, a little cramping. This is known as *mittelschmerz* (middle pain) because it comes at mid-cycle.

Although the egg is the largest cell in a woman's body, it is smaller than a grain of salt. When it is released from the follicle it drops into the reach of at the end of the fallopian tube. The inside of this tube, which is about the width of a hollow piece of spaghetti, is lined with hair-like projections (called cilia) which move the egg along. Special cells in the lining of the fallopian tube secrete a fluid that nourishes and helps to transport the sperm and eggs.

The fallopian tubes are the egg's route to the uterus (womb) but they are also the destination of any sperm which have been ejaculated into the woman's body. For a 'text book' conception, between 50 to 100 million sperm will have been deposited by the man high up in the woman's vagina. Some will die instantly but others will swim up the stream of the woman's 'fertile mucus', through the cervical canal (the pathway through the cervix), into the uterine cavity and from there into the fallopian tubes where they wait for the egg to happen along. During this journey the sperm undergo changes which 'prime' them, preparing them for fertilization.

While the egg is passing along the fallopian tubes towards the uterus, the empty follicle, which is now known as the *corpus luteum*, begins to release a new hormone, progesterone. This gives the endometrium a signal to prepare itself to receive a successfully fertilized egg. In response to the progesterone, the endometrium plumps itself up to provide a rich, nourishing environment. At the beginning of her cycle, a woman's endometrium may be just 0.5 mm thick, but by the time it is ready to receive a fertilized egg it will have increased it's thickness 14-fold to 7 mm.

The progesterone also instructs the cervix to halt its production of sperm-friendly mucus and start making a thicker mucus which will plug the cervical canal to prevent bacteria entering the cervix. It also orders the pituitary gland to halt its production of LH or FSH.

The surge in progesterone is responsible for some pre-menstrual symptoms such as breast swelling and tenderness, and bloatedness as well as some of the symptoms of early pregnancy (see pp. 28–32). This explains why some women often describe the early symptoms as being a continuation of those they usually get before a period: they are effectively the same symptoms caused by the same hormone.

(3) After ovulation—conception

The egg must be fertilized within 24 hours of its release. However, this does not mean that a woman can only become pregnant if she has sex in the day after ovulation. If a couple have had intercourse in the few days before ovulation, when the vaginal fluids are particularly sperm-friendly, it is possible for sperm to be already present in her fallopian tubes when the egg is released. Sperm can survive in the fallopian tubes for as long as five days, and some experts think that so-called 'super-sperm' can last for seven. This means that it is quite possible to become pregnant from an act of intercourse that took place a few days *before* ovulation.

When sperm encounter the egg they surround it and secrete enzymes that break down the egg's protective case. Although only one sperm will actually fertilize the egg, it takes a certain number of sperm surrounding it to create the right conditions for that one to penetrate. Once the head of one sperm penetrates the egg, a special mechanism is triggered which prevents other sperm from entering.

The woman's body soon identifies whether or not the egg has been fertilized. If fertilization has occurred, the egg, travelling along the fallopian tube to the uterus, sends a chemical signal to the corpus luteum instructing it to continue pumping out progesterone. If the egg is not fertilized, progesterone production stops, and in response to the decreased supply the womb lining begins to break down and the womb starts to contract to its pre-engorged size. The stored blood oozes away through the cervix and into the vagina as a menstrual period. As soon as the pituitary gland realizes that progesterone is no longer being produced, the whole cycle begins all over again.

As the early embryo begins to implant in the womb lining about seven days after fertilization, it begins to secrete human chorionic gonadotrophin (hCG). This is thought to influence the lining of the womb in such a way as to allow the embryo to attach itself and encourages the womb to maintain it.

The reaction of a woman's body to the developing embryo is quite unique. From the moment of fertilization the early embryo is distinct from other tissue in the woman's body. It has its own distinct genetic profile which, as 50 per cent is determined by the sperm, is different from that of the woman in which it resides.

Normal cells contain 46 chromosomes—tiny thread-like structures each of which carries about 2000 genes. The genes, in turn, carry a blueprint for inherited characteristics. Sperm and egg cells are distinct from all other cells in the human body in that they contain only half the usual number of chromosomes: just 23 each. This means that when the sperm fuses with the egg and fertilization takes place, chromosomes from the sperm and the egg pair up to make the full complement of 46. In the rare case that more than one sperm manages to enter the egg (a condition known as polyspermic fertilization) too much genetic material will be present. The embryo will have too many chromosomes and will probably spontaneously miscarry.

The fertilized egg contains one sex chromosome from the mother and one from the father. The mother's is always the same and is known as the X chromosome, while the sex chromosome from the sperm may be either an X or a Y chromosome. If the egg is fertilized by a sperm containing an X chromosome a female (XX) embryo will result. When the sperm contains a Y-chromosome the embryo will be male (XY).

The developing embryo is, in fact, a foreign body: a kind of parasite rather than a part of the woman's body. Usually when a human body detects that there is something alien within it, it mobilizes forces to eliminate the invader. The immune system triggers a barrage of search and destroy procedures to locate the outsider. This is why organ transplants often fail, and would always fail if special procedures were not followed to ensure that the recipient of any donated tissue is as close a match to the donor as possible, and special drugs were not given to suppress the 'search and destroy' response. With a developing embryo, the situation is entirely different. Right from the very start it interacts with the woman's body to create the most favourable conditions for itself.

The start of pregnancy

Although the very early embryo begins to affect the woman's body by producing hormone signals from the time of fertilization, 'pregnancy' as most people understand it does not really begin until slightly later.

Medically speaking, pregnancy is usually taken to begin *not* at the time of fertilization, but when the early embryo (known as a blastocyst) attaches itself in the uterus, usually between day 21 and 24 of a woman's cycle (counting from the first day of her last period). There are sound reasons for this distinction.

Although it is the case that the embryo has a distinct genetic profile, from the time that the genetic material carried by the sperm fuses with that of the egg it is still extremely uncertain whether it will develop. Research suggests that as many as one fertilized egg in four fails to implant in which case a woman would have her period as normal without even knowing that fertilization had taken place.

If pregnancy were defined as occurring at the point of fertilization it would have bizarre practical consequences. What would it mean, for example, for a couple undergoing *in vitro* fertilization treatment (IVF), in which eggs are fertilized outside the body and returned when they have shown themselves capable of development? It would be meaningless to describe a woman as pregnant when her embryo was still in a laboratory dish (or even a freezer if the fertilized eggs are to be cryopreserved for a later embryo transfer), and when she knew that a crucial part of the struggle to have a child, the transfer of the embryo to her womb and the wait to see if it would implant, was still to come.

The recognition that pregnancy begins at implantation is also important in distinguishing between abortion and contraception. Abortion is regarded as a measure which ends a pregnancy once it has begun whilst contraception prevents a pregnancy from taking place. Some methods of contraception work partly by altering conditions in the body to make it difficult for a fertilized egg to implant in the womb. For example the IUD is thought sometimes to prevent implantation and one of the effects of the progestogen-only contraceptive pill is to prevent the changes to the womb lining which make it hospitable to a fertilized egg. Emergency contraception also sometimes relies on preventing implantation.

Some people who insist that a new and sacrosanct human life is created at fertilization believe that such methods of contraception should be redefined as abortion, but this view has been rejected by the medical and legal establishment.

This issue is likely to a subject of much controversy in coming years as new methods of contraception are developed which clearly act to prevent implantation rather than fertilization—for example, a once-a-month pill.

Despite general agreement among the medical profession that a pregnancy begins at implantation, when a doctor in the UK or North America dates a *confirmed* pregnancy, he or she will calculate the length of the pregnancy from the first day of the woman's last menstrual period. This means that by the time that the period of a pregnant woman with a regular 28 day cycle is 2 weeks overdue, her doctor and those subsequently involved in the management of her pregnancy will consider her to be six weeks pregnant. This is the case despite the fact that implantation will probably only have taken place approximately three weeks previously and fertilization perhaps another five days before that.

Doctors date pregnancy in this way because it is the only significant date of which they can be absolutely certain. Most women ovulate at mid-cycle, but not all do and even if a woman generally has a regular cycle, it may be the case that the one cycle in which she conceived was the exception to the rule. Even if a woman is aware of exactly when she had the act of sex which led to the pregnancy, a doctor is not able to tell how long it was between the depositing of the sperm and fertilization.

Doctors in France and many other European countries work to a different convention and date pregnancies from mid-cycle. So a woman who is ten weeks pregnant in Paris is at the same stage of her pregnancy as a woman who is twelve weeks pregnant in London.

For the purposes of medical accuracy, pregnancy measured 'by date' or by 'last menstrual period (LMP)' refers to the amount of time from the first day of the last menstrual period. Pregnancy by 'gestation' refers to the time since the estimated date of conception which can be assessed fairly accurately once the size and stage of development of the embryo can be observed with an ultrasound scan (usually at around six weeks by LMP).

The way a woman relates to the developing embryo is usually shaped by the way she feels about the pregnancy in general. If the pregnancy is welcome she may already think of the embryo as a child (with a name and a personality) even before its body-parts are formed. On the other hand, if the pregnancy is resented and the woman has no intention of considering any alternative to abortion, she may see the embryo as nothing more than a problem which she wishes to resolve as soon as possible.

The subjective differences in how pregnancies are experienced helps to explain why so often women fail to understand each other's sentiments about pregnancy. A woman who has experienced a pregnancy as an invasion of her life and body and who is repulsed by the idea of having her partner's child has nothing in common with a woman eagerly anticipating a much loved and wanted baby, save their physical state. A woman with a wanted pregnancy may feel that she cannot understand how anyone could have an abortion. A woman with an unwanted pregnancy may just as sincerely fail to understand how anyone could want a baby.

Many women looking forward to a second 'wanted' pregnancy, having aborted a former unwanted pregnancy, remark on how entirely different they feel.

No one can tell you how you will feel, or how you should feel when you are pregnant. It depends on a complex cocktail of factors, only some of which are biological. Pregnancy is a state of mind as well as a state of body. Your feelings play as much a part as your hormones.

References

1. Sheila Kitzinger (1992). *The new pregnancy and childbirth*, p. 33. Michael Joseph, London.
2. Institute of Population Studies (1993). *Sexual health and family planning services in general practice: Report of a qualitative research survey in England and Wales*. Family Planning Association, London.

3
Making choices

The decision to end a pregnancy occurs in an entirely different emotional context to that of 'trying for a child'. Terminating a pregnancy is not the same as never having started it.

The decision of a woman or a couple to have a baby can evolve gradually. She may decide that she would like a child some time in the future—but not now. Next she may change her method of contraception, perhaps from a hormonal to a barrier method, to allow her body to establish its natural cycle. Then she may begin to alter her life to prepare her body and mind for her future condition by starting to take the recommended vitamin supplements, by giving up smoking, and taking up exercise to tone her muscles. She and her partner may have discussions to plan the most convenient time for her to be pregnant. At all times the situation can be renegotiated: minds can change, and conception can be delayed. Some couples spend their whole fertile lives deferring the decision because the time is never quite right.

If a woman becomes pregnant accidentally, however, the terms of the discussion change entirely. Instead of having deliberately to set the pregnancy process in motion, she has consciously to decide to end it. The terms of the *status quo* change. Before, she may well have thought her existing life-style would continue indefinitely; once pregnant to continue as she is means that her life will change utterly. If she does not arrange an abortion she will face either first-time motherhood, or an addition to the family, in a matter of months. Many women describe the feeling as 'like being on a roller coaster' or a 'conveyer belt'. Suddenly her body not only *feels* out of her control, but *is* out of her control, and this can be very disturbing.

For some women the decision about an unplanned pregnancy is straightforward: they want to end it as quickly as possible, put the experience behind them, and get on with their lives. For others, it will be equally straightforward in that the pregnancy will be a delightful surprise. It is a myth that *all* women will find the decisions about unplanned pregnancy difficult, although most probably do and many women are surprised at the difficulty they have over what they previously thought would be a straightforward issue.

All women with accidental pregnancies—even those with a clear cut and uncomplicated idea of what they want—have to confront feelings about the potential baby and about their own fertility, life-style, and relationships.

Mixed feelings

There are many reasons why women have ambivalent feelings towards their situation.

An unplanned pregnancy can deliver a severe blow to a woman's confidence, especially if her self-esteem is built upon her ability to control her life. As Chapter 1 outlines, accidental pregnancies happen even to women who have been meticulous about their con-traception and made every reasonable effort to prevent pregnancy. When you become pregnant in these conditions it can generate intense feelings of **self-doubt**—if your fertility, your body, is out of control, what does it say about the rest of your life?

The situation can be particularly disturbing if a woman has pre-viously felt unsympathetic towards other women in this predicament. Despite publicity about contraceptive failure rates and broader discus-sions about the reasons for unplanned pregnancy, there is still a prevail-ing sentiment in society that it is the consequence of carelessness or fickle behaviour. Women who are in 'controlling' positions at work, or who like to project an image of infallibility, may feel particularly humili-ated and undermined by the experience. The reaction of Rose, a family planning nurse, to her unplanned pregnancy is one that may be shared by many whose work presupposes some kind of medical knowledge.

'It was really difficult to admit to myself that I had been caught, and it was absolutely impossible for me to admit it to any of my colleagues given the amount of time we spent joking about the girls who come into the clinic. I felt so shaken up, and so stupid—especially because the day after I had unprotected sex I thought about getting the morn-ing-after pill but I decided against it. I kept thinking it was all so unlike me there had to be a reason—like perhaps it was nature telling me something. Eventually I came to my senses and realized I was trying to make excuses to myself for what is, after all, a really common slip-up. It made me face one fact: I was no better and no worse than anyone else who takes a chance and doesn't get away with it.'

Placed in a situation where it seems (even if this is not the case) as though her judgement, self-control, or self-reliance has failed her, a woman may doubt her ability to make decisions about, or plan for, anything. If she has a strong sense of her own rationality, she may wonder if there is some, perhaps subconscious, reason why she has allowed the pregnancy to happen. Consequently she may feel confused and unclear about which path she should follow.

Sometimes the **confirmation of fertility** may be a relief, even though a woman is distressed about the pregnancy itself. It is only on becoming pregnant that a woman *knows* for certain that she is fertile. Until that time she may have assumed this, but there has always been room for doubt.

In recent years the issues of subfertility and infertility have achieved a particularly high profile in the media. In an attempt to take away the stigma of infertility, health promotion agencies, such as the Family Planning Association and the Health Education Authority have sought to normalize it by stressing the high proportion of couples who have problems. Furthermore, as new infertility treatments and techniques have become available, service providers have sought to promote them by emphasizing the number of couples who may be able to take advantage of them. The growing public awareness of infertility is a development that has greatly benefited those who suffer from fertility problems, but it may have had an unintended effect of generating unnecessary anxiety in many who do not. For example, it is no longer uncommon for teenagers seeking family planning advice to express doubts about their fertility—especially if they know they have had unprotected sex from which they have not conceived. Some womens' health clinics report an increase in the number of women enquiring about 'fertility screening' to confirm that they are potentially able to have a child.

There are few women who are indifferent to their fertility. Even if a woman is certain that she never wants a child, she wants it to be by *choice*, and not because she cannot have one. Consequently the confirmation of a pregnancy, however unwelcome at that particular moment, can be a relief. It is a confirmation that she is ovulating, producing the correct hormones in the right amount and that her womb is capable of sustaining a pregnancy. This may generate many positive feelings about the pregnancy despite the fact that she is sure that she does not want the child that will result.

Cindy's reaction, when she was 18, to her accidental pregnancy is extremely common:

> 'I felt such a strange mixture of emotions when the test showed I was pregnant. I felt very frightened; I hadn't a clue what I was going to do. It was my worst dream come true. But at the same time I couldn't help feeling a bit proud of myself. It was real evidence that I was a woman, and my body was doing what nature intended.'

These seemingly contradictory feelings can even be present in women who have conceived as a consequence of assisted conception. For a sub-fertile couple, many years of tests and treatments may be needed to achieve a pregnancy. During that time the lives of both partners may have been focused on achieving a viable pregnancy, and they may not have allowed themselves to consider beyond that point. This means that when a pregnancy is established they are confronted for the first time with the same set of doubts that worry couples who have conceived without medical intervention. If many years have passed between the start of treatment and the start of a pregnancy, it may even be the case that the reasons which compelled them to join an infertility programme are no longer pressing. For the first time they may feel able to ask themselves: 'Do we really want this?'. And the answer may be, 'No'.

There are many women who, in the abstract, would love to have a child but are unable to welcome a pregnancy at the time it occurs. This situation can be particularly difficult for the woman as she may find that people are relatively unsympathetic to her plight and expect her to reorganize her life around the pregnancy in spite of the fact that this may not be acceptable or even possible.

A woman whose pregnancy occurs at the **'wrong time'** is particularly susceptible to the judgemental attitudes of others, including many doctors who, when faced with a woman 'who wants a child at some time but not now', are inclined to weigh up whether or not *they* think the timing of the pregnancy is appropriate. Thus it is often assumed that an abortion is the most sensible option for a pregnant 15-year-old, even if motherhood is her main ambition, while a married, childless 30-year-old may be expected to 'come to terms' with having a child. So, a doctor writing in the *British Medical Journal*[1] to justify her refusal to refer a woman for an abortion because she felt that the reason for the woman's request (that the pregnancy would disrupt her skiing holiday) was trivial, solicited a chorus of approval. The case was reported in the national press and has since been used, by the anti-choice lobby, as a notorious example of the alleged 'fecklessness' of some women. Even some pro-choice campaigners felt unable to support this particular woman's right to choose to end her unwanted pregnancy. The request for the abortion was seen to be particularly offensive because the woman was honest about the fact that she wished to conceive again at some time in the near future.

Although for some women timing can turn a potentially wanted pregnancy into one that is unwanted, for others the situation can be much more ambiguous. For example, a pregnancy that occurs as little as one month before it was planned can disqualify a woman from maternity leave and the right to resume her job. A mis-timed conception could cause disastrous disruptions to a student's exams or to a business woman's career. Situations such as these can be particularly difficult to resolve because the feelings towards the pregnancy may be, in the main, positive despite the fact that the woman concerned can only continue the pregnancy at considerable disadvantage to herself. A woman faced with a strong desire to have her baby, but who feels that circumstances make it impossible for her to consider that option, is particularly emotionally vulnerable, as Phillipa discovered:

'I desperately wanted the baby but if I hadn't had the abortion I would have lost my job and that would have been the end of everything because we were already behind on the mortgage. Peter couldn't understand why I couldn't explain to my boss, but he doesn't understand how cut-throat the consultancy world is. You are paid well, but you're expected to organize your personal life around your contracts. It's hard enough for a woman anyway, but if I had announced that I would not be able to run the most prestigious project we had ever won because I would be on maternity leave when the main conference was scheduled . . . I would have been finished.
I think I went into shock at the time of abortion. I felt so numb. Then I really freaked out. I ended up on valium for two weeks.'

Sometimes a pregnancy can be at the right time but by the **wrong partner**. One of the qualities that makes us distinct from the rest of the animal kingdom is our conscious use of sex for recreation as well as procreation. A woman may find a man sexually desirable without wishing him to be the father of her child. Thus is it perfectly possible and, indeed quite common, for a woman to wish to have a child (even to have one now), but not by her current sexual partner.

This can lead to a great deal of angst particularly if the pregnancy has occurred as a consequence of a liaison with a man who is not the woman's regular sexual partner, perhaps as a result of an affair, or a 'one-night stand'. If others know of the pregnancy, the woman's true feelings may contradict those that all those around her expect her to have. Her family and friends may expect her to be delighted while she is filled with dread that she may be found out.

A woman in this position has to consider just how much about the circumstances of the conception she wishes to explain to her regular partner. Should she allow him to think that he is responsible? If she keeps her affair secret and she has the child, will she be found out? The expanding range of genetic tests, and the emphasis on the importance of knowledge about one's genetic history mean that it is far more difficult to ensure that the 'guilty secrets', which in the past would remain secret as long as the urge to confess was resisted, are no longer secure. Barbara, pregnant by a casual lover, describes her situation as 'sheer hell'.

'I had to lie and tell my husband that my sister was ill and needed me to stay—just to get some time away from him so I could think. Every situation seemed impossible. I couldn't imagine how I could have an abortion without him knowing, yet if I had the kid I would be living a lie for the rest of my life. There was no way I could explain to [her husband] what had happened. There would have been no argument—he would have left me, and I really loved him . . .

. . . in the end I arranged to have the abortion in London and told him I had to see a specialist because I had got some gynaecological problem. That was how I explained the vomiting. He was really sympathetic and that made me feel even worse.'

Many doctors involved in infertility treatment have anecdotes of women who have become pregnant by a lover while participating in treatment to overcome a problem with their partner's sperm. The strains on a woman in this situation are enormous as she may feel that the conflict between her desire to become a mother and her desire to maintain her relationship with an infertile partner is irre-solvable.

For a woman approaching the end of her fertile years, an un-expected pregnancy may present a 'last chance' for a child. This sentiment is as likely to be experienced by a woman who has already had children as it is by one who is pregnant for the first time.

A woman who has never conceived may be acutely aware that the option of motherhood is quickly closing. Although there has been considerable public discussion of the potential of new reproductive technologies to override the menopause and push back the age at which women can bear children, most women are aware that these techniques will not be of benefit to them directly. A woman approaching 40 knows that she has only a few years in which she is able to exercise the choice to be a mother. This places particular pressure on women who do not have a partner or who are in rela-tionship with a man who does not wish to have children.

A woman who becomes pregnant towards the end of her fertile years may be unhappy about the circumstances of the pregnancy, or about her choice of partner, or the exact timing, but nevertheless welcome the opportunity to be a mother. Even if she decides to end the pregnancy by abortion she may be pleased that she has been able to reaffirm to herself that she is childless by choice rather than by force of circumstance. Sheila, accidentally pregnant at 43 found:

> 'In a bizarre way I was pleased it happened. There was no real ques-tion of me having the child, although I dithered about it for a week. But I was pleased I had been able to get pregnant. I had always won-dered what it felt like, and now I knew. There was one night where I sat up thinking: "If you don't do it now you'll never have a chance again". I told myself I had to have the abortion because of the risk of handicap, but I think that was just my excuse to myself to stop me being in such turmoil about it.'

A woman who regarded her family as complete may also have mixed feelings about a surprise pregnancy because it represents a chance to step back into a phase of her life that she thought was gone forever. This may particularly be the case if her existing children have passed puberty and are known to be sexually active. A woman in this situation may feel that she is moving into the 'grandmother' generation—a feeling that may sit uncomfortably with the image she has of herself. Sally, pregnant as a result of a split condom found that:

'For a moment I was elated, I think I actually punched the air! I had thought my missed period was the start of my menopause. I only did the pregnancy test because I had read an article about women who put their pregnancy symptoms down to something else. I was really keen to go for it, but [her husband] went up the wall. He said there was no way he was starting again. And of course he was right. It would have been really stupid.'

Often older women's feelings about an unplanned pregnancy may be complicated by their fear of the increased risks of fetal abnormality. By the time she is 40, a woman's risk of bearing a child with Down's syndrome is one in 100, compared to a risk of less than one in 1000 from women in their twenties. Many genetic problems can be detected through antenatal screening techniques but some women who would otherwise have welcomed a pregnancy feel that the possible risk of disability is too great.

Life is unpredictable and our **circumstances change**. This means it is quite possible for a pregnancy that was originally planned and wanted may be subsequently perceived as a disaster. This is particularly true in times of economic insecurity when, for many, extreme financial hardship, even the threat of homelessness, can strike couples who thought their lives were stable and their livelihood secure. Redundancy, wage cuts, or the calling in of a loan can create the circumstances where a couple feel it is impossible to continue with even a much-wanted and planned pregnancy.

Changes in a relationship can also change the way a woman feels about pregnancy. Three weeks after she had found out that she was pregnant, Jackie found out that her husband, a university lecturer, had been having an affair with one of his students.

'I would not have believed my feelings could change so quickly. I was so repulsed, by him and by the idea of his baby inside me. It was so sordid. He had been discussing plans for the nursery with me and then going off to screw her. Everything seemed like a complete sham. I couldn't believe I had been so taken in. Suddenly I loathed him, and because of that I loathed the baby too. When I saw the counsellor at the clinic she asked me if I might be having the abortion to get back at him. Maybe there was something of that in it, but mainly it was because I just fell out of love with the baby when I fell out of love with him.'

Sometimes the announcement of a pregnancy can cause a crisis in a relationship, particularly if it is unexpected. Just as a woman has to consider the responsibilities of motherhood, so a man has to consider his role as a potential father. Many men find this extremely unsettling, even if they have previously expressed a wish to have children at some time. Today, for many couples, starting a family has assumed the role that the marriage ceremony played 20 years ago: it is seen as an expression of permanent commitment. Consequently an accidental pregnancy can force on to the agenda an appraisal of a joint future that may have remained undiscussed to this point.

A woman's attitude to her pregnancy can be significantly shaped by her partner's attitude towards her. A woman may have initially welcomed a pregnancy but if her partner is unenthusiastic, it may alter how she feels about both the pregnancy and herself.

Ultimately the decision about the future of a pregnancy rests with the woman. However, most women know that making a choice which is deeply resented by her partner risks undermining their relationship. **Conflicts may occur** about a pregnancy just as they occur about every other area of life. This can be the case whatever decision she makes: a man may strongly object to his partner having an abortion, or he may just as strongly object to her having 'his' child. By making men financially responsible for their offspring the Child Support Act 1993 may unfortunately have added to the pressures on a woman to terminate a pregnancy that her partner does not want.

An unplanned pregnancy may bring all manner of pre-existing tensions in a relationship to the surface. The decision cannot be left unresolved, nor even deferred indefinitely and the situation may reveal that both partners have different expectations of the relationship and their future lives. Susie found that:

'We started off discussing what we should do about the baby and ended up discussing what we should do about our lives. The more we talked it became clear that we both wanted really different things. I wanted to settle down, and I had assumed that was what Nick wanted, but he announced he wanted to go on the road with another band.'

Conflict with other family members can be equally traumatic. A young woman living at home with her parents may feel particularly frightened and confused—especially if she is still dependent on her parents and so under their control. It is unlikely that a young woman who is economically dependent on her parents will be able to make a decision about her pregnancy which is entirely independent of their concerns. If she has her baby, her parents will almost inevitably be drawn into caring for the child while if she opts for an abortion she may need their financial help.

Inter-generational conflicts over the future of a pregnancy can also occur when existing children make their views known. The possibility of a new addition to the family can provoke intensely strong feelings from existing children, who may have all manners of fears— rational and irrational. This is particularly the case when children are adolescent and asserting their independence from their parents. They may have difficulty in coming to terms with the evidence that their parents are still sexually active, or they may feel that the stability of the family unit is being undermined. Joan, pregnant at 43 and with children aged 20 and 16 was upset to find

'The kids were horrified. [My eldest] even gave me a leaflet for some abortion clinic and tried to talk to me about how I shouldn't feel guilty about wanting an abortion. But I *didn't* want an abortion, and [her husband] didn't want me to have one either. We were thrilled but they seemed really disgusted.

'I couldn't work out if it was because they felt it would have a big effect on them, or if they were worried about me. But it really brought me down, and I did wonder if I was being really selfish. Fortunately my doctor was brilliant and backed me all the way. He said he thought the kids were being selfish little brats'.

Conflicts may be particularly intense if a new baby will in some way compromise the living or social arrangements of the existing children, for example if holidays have to be cancelled or bedrooms shared. Conflicts can also occur if a woman decides to terminate the pregnancy, but her children have a moral objection to abortion.

The attitude of friends and colleagues can also influence a woman's feelings about her pregnancy. We tend to seek out and associate with other like-minded people who share our values, priorities, and who have a similar life-styles. Childless couples often tend to associate with other childless couples, and share a common freedom from the ties of family life. This common interest of such a friendship group may be undermined when one of the group declares their intention to have a child. Annie described the reaction of a close friend to her surprise pregnancy.

'Peter and I were delighted when the pregnancy was confirmed; although we'd always said we didn't want kids, I think both of us had gradually come round to the idea. It never occurred to either of us that our friends would be anything other than delighted. We had a pretty close relationship with two other couples—we went on holiday together, spent Christmases together, shared the same taste in music, films, and food. Dinner parties were a big part of our social life.

'In fact, we had planned to announce that I was pregnant over dinner one evening once I got to 12 weeks, but it didn't work out like that because Janet cornered me and asked me outright if I was and so we had to admit it.

'Of course, everyone *said* they were happy for us, but you would have had to be totally insensitive not to have picked up all the signals. It was as though we had changed the rules of the game, and in a way we had. We wouldn't be skiing this year, if they came to us as usual at Christmas there would be a child to contend with. We had to start to watch our spending for the first time. I had to make a real effort not to talk about morning sickness, stretch marks, and birthing plans, and that felt strange; for the first time my concerns were entirely different to those of my best friends.

'I remember feeling really down, about 16 weeks into the pregnancy, and thinking I hadn't bargained for this. I had thought a baby would be an addition to our life, but I realized that it meant more sacrifices than I had ever imagined. For a moment I really did wonder if I was ready to make them.'

One of the most difficult situations for a woman to be in is when her feelings about her own pregnancy conflict with her **moral beliefs**.

In general, attitudes to abortion tend to be shaped by abstract considerations. The questions posed are usually those such as: when does life begin? do fetuses have rights? is the fetus a person and if so at what stage does it become one? The perspective of the woman, for whom the pregnancy has intense practical consequences, is often left off the agenda. However, when a woman is confronted by her own unplanned pregnancy, the questions she asks herself tend to be of a more personal and pragmatic nature such as: how will *I* cope? what consequences will this have for *my* life?

Bernie has been on marches against abortion but she says she was appalled to find that:

> 'There was a time when I did consider it. When my third was just six months I fell pregnant again. The doctor said he didn't think I could cope because I had been very bad with my blood pressure the last time and I still wasn't right. I did have a long hard think. I couldn't, in my heart, welcome this baby and I had responsibilities to my three. I prayed so hard for deliverance, and I had a miscarriage. The doctors says it was because my body wasn't ready to cope, but I believe it was Jesus saving me from sin.'

Choices such as adoption, which may in theory have seemed feasible practical alternatives to abortion, may not be appropriate to the particular circumstances of *this* pregnancy—if, for example, it is important that the pregnancy remains a secret.

A woman facing this kind of moral conflict may feel particularly confused and isolated. She may feel appalled that she is able to consider a course of action which she believes to be morally repugnant, or she may feel that her entire system of values and beliefs is called into question.

When choices narrow

An unplanned pregnancy poses a practical problem which requires an equally practical solution. *In practice* the choices that are available may not be as wide as they might seem *in principle*. This book considers three courses of action: abortion, adoption, and motherhood. If you are pregnant you will inevitably end up following one of these. But prevailing circumstances may force you into a decision you would rather not have made.

Many women are sufficiently self-reliant and determined to swim against the stream and either keep their baby, or have an abortion, in the face of tremendous opposition. Each year several thousand women cross the Irish Sea to have abortions in Britain because they cannot end their pregnancies in this way in their own country. Often these journeys are undertaken in conditions of utter secrecy. On the other hand, there are young women who, despite pressure to terminate the pregnancy or to give up their child for adoption, insist on raising their baby and do so just as well as older women with planned pregnancies.

But, however inventive, resourceful, and determined a woman might be, she may find herself in circumstances where she feels there really is only one course of action. Indeed, there may only be one option open to her.

It is important to consider all the 'theoretical options' even if you reject them in the end. Whatever decision you make there will probably be times when you will wonder what would have happened if you had made a different choice. By considering your theoretical options now, though, you may find that in the future you can be confident that you made the right decision.

What ever you decide, there are certain facts that you have to face up to:

- *There is no going back*
  You cannot put the clock back and become 'unpregnant' again. And, once you have committed yourself to a course of action, there will come a point when you cannot change your mind. If you decide on abortion you can change your mind at any time until the procedure actually starts. In the case of adoption you can change your mind at any time before the final papers are signed.

- *You did not want to be in this situation*
  But you are, and there is no point in blaming yourself or those around you. You will probably have 'if-only-this-had-never-happened' or 'why me?' thoughts, but this is a very unproductive way to think and keeps you trapped in the past when you need to think about the future. Try to draw an imaginary line under what has happened in the past and plan what you need to do from *now*.

- *You need to take control*
  You may feel that your body has rebelled against you and your life is careering out of control. In a way it has and it is. But that does not mean it has to stay that way. There *are* things you can do and decisions you can take to put yourself back on the right road.

- *There is a solution to the problem*
  An unplanned pregnancy is a resolvable problem. There are things that you can do to alter your situation.

- *You are the only person who can decide what is best for you*
  No one else can know *exactly* how you feel about your situation. Your feelings about the pregnancy are vitally important because they will shape how you will cope after you have made your decision. It may help to discuss how you feel and seek advice from others, but ultimately *you* have to live with the consequences of your decision. Only you know with what you can and cannot cope. What seems right for someone else may not be right for you.

- *You can and will make the right decision*
  Serious decisions are frightening. They are seldom completely straightforward and so we worry about making a mistake. It helps to remember that no one is more able than you to make the right decision, and you need to trust yourself to make it. Try to be confident about yourself.

It may help to:

- *Take time to think about your situation*
  If you think you will decide to have an abortion you will need to make up your mind quite quickly, but even then you can give yourself several days to consider your options. It is important to find out how long you have been pregnant, because this may have important practical implications. If you are more than ten weeks pregnant you may find it more difficult to get an abortion if you do not set the wheels in motion soon. A doctor will be able to give you a fairly accurate estimate. If you do not want to consult your own doctor you can see another doctor in another general practice, a family planning clinic, or young persons clinic. Try not to panic.

You my want to put off thinking about your problem, and it is easy to come up with all kinds of reasons why you can't face thinking about it now, but you will tomorrow. Try not to keep putting it off. This is one problem that will not go away if you don't think about it. It may help to fix a 'thinking and decision' time.

- *Decide who you want to tell and who you want to discuss things with*
  You may find it helps to discuss your situation with your partner, your family, or your friends. Or you may prefer to talk to someone who will be more detached, professional, and who will not breach your confidence. Your doctor may a good person with whom to discuss your options, or you can see a counsellor at a family planning clinic, Brook Advisory Centre, a pregnancy advisory service, or women's health clinic. The not-for-profit agencies which provide abortion services (British Pregnancy Advisory Service, Pregnancy Advisory Service and Marie Stopes Clinics) offer counselling that is genuinely non-directive, which means they will not try to encourage you to have an abortion or to continue the pregnancy but will help you to explore your own feelings. Life (the agency) also offers counselling but they will not provide information about abortion.

- *Decide what information you need*
  The more you know about your options, the more in control you will be. You may find that some of the ideas you had about a particular course of action were wrong and that knowing the facts allows you to consider an option you would have previously dismissed. For example, if you believe an abortion will damage your health you may not even consider it as an option, but on finding that it is a very safe operation may write it back on to your agenda. The same goes for adoption or having your child. You may think you could never have a child adopted because you have very out-of-date ideas about adoption, or you may not realize the practical support available to single mothers. Often it is not until we are in a situation that we discover the real facts of the matter.

Whose decision?

Only in very exceptional circumstances can a woman's decision about her pregnancy be interfered with.

Father's rights

Abortion law in Britain does not insist that the father of the fetus should be consulted, or even notified, and he certainly has no right of veto over the woman's actions. The position is clearer than in North America or many European countries because abortion is understood to be a medical issue rather than a matter of individual rights. For an abortion to be legal in Britain, the medical profession must concede that the continuance of the pregnancy would be problematic for the woman or her family (see Chapter 4, pp. 69–72). This third party endorsement means that the issue is not susceptible to the kind of debates that takes place in, for example, the USA, where men have argued that their right to have the child is as valid as the woman's right not to have it.

Various attempts have been made by men, in the UK to prevent women from aborting pregnancies which they have fathered, but these have always failed. In 1979, a husband took a case to the European Commission of Human Rights following the refusal of the English courts to grant him an injunction to prevent his wife from terminating her pregnancy. The case was thrown out because the abortion was certified as necessary for the woman's health. The most well-known English case involved a student at Oxford University who sought to prevent his girlfriend from having an abortion in 1982. This also failed, although the woman was so traumatized by the experience of the legal battle that she decided to have the child anyway.

It seems to be generally accepted in legal circles that the claimed rights of putative fathers, when they come into conflict with the desires of pregnant women, are too difficult to enforce in law, even if it were desirable to do so. In the 1979 case, which became known as *Paton v. Trustees of BPAS*[3], the court refused to contemplate enforcing 'supposed matrimonial obligations' when this might require the imprisonment of the woman. The ultimate futility in granting such an injunction in favour of a putative father was demonstrated in Canada where, in 1990, a man did obtain such a ruling. The court, in the predominantly Catholic state of Quebec, based its ruling on the right to life of the fetus, and also on the rights of the father, claiming that the fetus was 'his child as much as it is the mother's, neither more, neither less.'[3] However, the woman went ahead with the abortion anyway, making a mockery of the decision.

Parents' rights over young people

It is not strictly necessary for a young woman under the age of 16 to get permission to have an abortion from one or both of her parents, although parental consent makes things much easier for the medical staff involved, and they will always do their utmost to persuade her to inform her parents.

If a pregnant woman under the age of 16 seeks advice about abortion and refuses to involve her parents and guardians, despite her doctor's attempts to persuade her to do so, most hospitals will encourage her to involve another adult whom she feels she can trust, perhaps a teacher or family friend. Usually a social worker will be involved by the hospital, and the young girl will be carefully counselled to establish that she understands the consequences of her decision and is capable of giving her consent.

In the UK, the Children's Act clearly establishes that young people do have the right to give consent to medical treatment, which includes contraception and abortion, regardless of their age, providing they are capable of understanding the situation they are in. This principle had been ascertained earlier in case law when Lord Frazer, ruling in an appeal to the House of Lords brought by family values campaigner, Victoria Gillick, stated that: 'provided the patient, whether a boy or girl, is capable of understanding what is proposed, and of expressing his or her wishes, I see no good reason for holding that he or she lacks the capacity to express them validly and effect-ively and to authorise the medical man to make the examination or give the treatment which he advises.'[4] Lord Frazer was ruling in re-lation to whether a doctor should be able to prescribe contraception to a girl under the age of 16, but his ruling holds good for all medical treatment including abortion.

Young people also have the same right to confidentiality as adults—although, as with adults, a doctor can breach confidentiality if he or she believes it is essential to the well-being of the patient. If a doctor does intend to breach confidentiality then he or she must inform the young person beforehand. A doctor might feel he or she must breach confidentiality if the pregnancy was the result of incest, or if the young girl was being abused by an adult in authority such as a teacher.

Very few abortions are carried out on young girls without parental involvement. Even if a girl initially insists that she will not involve them, her reluctance may be overcome when she realizes that there are social workers and counsellors who will help her to deal with the problem, perhaps by being with her when she explains her situation to them.

Occasionally a young girl may refuse to involve her parents because they are vociferous in their opposition to abortion, and in these cases it often helps for a doctor to explain to them why he or she thinks it is in the girl's best interest for the pregnancy to be terminated. Sometimes parents have misconceptions about the safety of the operation.

Neither parents nor any state agency can force a woman to end a pregnancy that she wishes to continue, except in the rare case where she is judged to be incapable of understanding the consequences of her refusal. This might be the situation if she has a severe learning disability. These cases are often grey areas of the law. Most authorities seem to accept that if a woman is capable of understanding that she is pregnant, and what child birth and abortion means, then she is competent to give her own consent to an abortion or to choose to have her baby.

The rights of state agencies

A woman cannot choose to have an abortion if her reasons for wanting to end the pregnancy fall outside the terms of the current abortion law. This sounds very absolute, but in practice—because a doctor can take into account a woman's mental state and living conditions when assessing whether it will be a problem for her to continue the pregnancy—things are rather more flexible. This is discussed at length in the next chapter.

State agencies can prevent a woman from deciding to keep her child if they feel that such a situation would place the child at risk. Thus a pregnant woman who has been convicted of child abuse or neglect may find that her child will be made a ward of court from the time that it is born.

For the vast majority of women the decisions about an unplanned pregnancy are *hers*. The next three chapters outline what each of the options involve.

References

1. Greenhalgh, T. (1992). 'A doctor's right to choose'. *British Medical Journal*, **305**, 371.
2. [1979] Q.B. 278. Discussed in Gillian Douglas (1991). *Law, fertility and reproduction* pp. 82–83. Sweet and Maxwell, London.
3. Discussed in G. Marshall (1988). *Liberty, abortion, and constitutional review in Canada*, Public Law, **199**.
4. Case of Gillick v. West Norfolk and Wisbech Area Health Authority [1986] discussed in Brenda M. Hoggett and David S. Pearl (1991). *The family, law and society*, Butterworths, London.

4

Considering abortion

No woman *wants* to have an abortion any more than she wants to have any other kind of operation. But just as a tonsillectomy may be considered the best solution for a woman with badly infected tonsils, so for some women an abortion may seem to be the best solution to an unplanned pregnancy. For some women the decision to end an unplanned pregnancy flies in the face of deeply held beliefs and principles, yet they may still feel it to be the only acceptable solution to their personal situation. Few women decide to have an abortion lightly. Even those women who find the very idea of motherhood appalling tend to think again when they discover they are pregnant. After all, most of us grow up believing we are destined to be mothers eventually, and many women take a certain pride in knowing that they are capable of motherhood—even if they do not wish to exercise their capacity for it now.

In Britain, one in five pregnancies—around 200 000 every year—end in abortion. There is no 'typical' woman who follows this road. The number includes women from every age, race, job, and social background. Official statistics[1] show that more women in their early 20s have abortions than those of other ages, but that is partly because there are more pregnancies in women in their early 20s than in any other age group.

A pregnant woman is more likely to have an abortion if she is single—even if she is cohabiting with her partner—than if she is married. Around 8 per cent of conceptions to married women end in abortion, compared to a third of conceptions outside marriage, but it must be remembered that because married women are much more likely to become pregnant than single women, they still account for almost a quarter of women having abortions.

The large number of abortions and the high abortion rate are often described as 'problems', especially by the media who find it an ideal issue to sensationalize. But abortion in itself is not the problem, rather the problem lies in the number of unplanned pregnancies. If fewer women had accidental pregnancies then fewer abortions would be needed.

The circumstances in which women live are a major influence in deciding whether to continue a pregnancy or choose to end it in abortion—and socio-economic status is a significant factor. Undoubtedly some economically disadvantaged women opt to end pregnancies because they feel that neither they, nor their family, could afford a child. But more usually, studies show the relationship between affluence and a woman's decision about her pregnancy is the other way round. A recent study of teenagers in Tayside in the North of England[2] showed that pregnant teenagers from 'affluent homes' are more likely to terminate their pregnancies than teenagers from 'deprived homes'. This may be because being pregnant and having a child gives such girls status in their families and communities and may seem to be the only emotionally rewarding activity available to them, even though the need to care for a child may increase their financial and housing problems. Girls from affluent homes, on the other hand, lose status by becoming pregnant and may have ambitious plans to continue their education which would be thwarted by motherhood. However, it would be wrong to assume from this that abortion is a middle-class option. The Tayside study shows that, among teenagers, those from deprived home are six times more likely to have an unplanned pregnancy—so teenagers from working-class backgrounds account for greater numbers of abortions. Similar studies of older women have not been made but in a recent publication by the Birth Control Trust, David Paintin argues that 'nationally, there are high correlations between factors associated with deprivation . . . and district abortion rates.'[3]

Having surveyed vast numbers of reports on unplanned pregnancy, the Royal College of Obstetricians and Gynaecologists concluded that a pregnancy was particularly likely to end in abortion 'if it would force the woman to abandon her plans for herself, or if she lacks the income, housing and personal support that she needs to cope with a child'.[4]

Looked at in this way it is possible to see the abortion 'option' as a positive and responsible choice made by a woman to put her back in charge of her life at a time when it seems to be slipping out of control.

Abortion is often seen as a moral or political issue rather than an issue of medical care and this may make it more difficult for women with unwanted pregnancies to find straightforward and honest answers to their questions. This chapter provides accurate information about abortion that any woman considering this option needs to know.

What is an abortion?

Abortion is a procedure carried out on a pregnant woman that terminates an existing pregnancy before what is known as 'viability' (the time when the child could be born and remain alive). It differs from contraception, which prevents a pregnancy from being established in the first place.

This definition is important because from time to time it has been claimed that emergency contraception is a form of abortion simply because it takes place after sex. What defines emergency contraception as 'contraception' is the fact that it prevents a pregnancy from being established in the first place. Although some people believe that the life of a new child begins at conception, when the egg is fertilized, the accepted medical and legal view is that a woman is not pregnant until the fertilized egg has implanted in her uterus.

When the 'older' pregnancy tests were in use which could not detect a pregnancy until the woman was two weeks late with her period, there would be a short period of time when it was impossible to confirm whether a woman was pregnant or not. Curiously, doctors could not conduct a legal abortion until they were able to confirm the existence of a pregnancy. Some would insist that the woman returned for a pregnancy test at a slightly later date, others would use the opportunity to carry out procedures to induce a 'menstrual period' without falling under the remit of the law.

In recent years there has been little room for doubt and any doctor carrying out a menstrual extraction procedure would find it impossible to argue that he or she had acted in 'good faith' believing that the woman was not pregnant, if a modern pregnancy test had not been carried out.

The law

Many people are surprised to find that British abortion law does not allow abortion on request at any stage in pregnancy. Nor is it the case, as in almost all other medical procedures, that the matter is simply left to the a doctor's clinical judgement. The circumstances in which a doctor can refer a woman for abortion are laid down in the 1967 Abortion Act which came into effect on 27 April 1968, and was slightly amended in 1991. The law in Britain insists that abortion is only legal if the conditions discussed below are met.

The abortion must be carried out by a registered medical practitioner and, except in an emergency, it must be carried out in either a National Health Service hospital or in a place that has been specially approved and registered by the Department of Health. Most non-NHS abortions take place in special charitable clinics run by the British Pregnancy Advisory Service (BPAS) and Marie Stopes Clinics, both of which have clinics throughout the country, or the Pregnancy Advisory Service (PAS) which is London-based. This network of non-profit making clinics was set up shortly after abortion was legalized, when it became clear that the NHS could not cope with the demand.

The provision of abortion on the National Health Service is still inadequate to the needs of women in England and Wales, providing only just over half of the abortions needed.[5] In Scotland the situation is far better with NHS services managing to provide more than 90 per cent of abortions. Those women in Scotland who have abortions in the private sector probably do so from choice rather than necessity. In England and Wales, research conducted by the PAS and BPAS show that the vast majority of women attending their clinics would have preferred an NHS abortion had they been able to arrange one.

All non-NHS clinics are regularly inspected by the Department of Health to ensure they conform to stringent standards.

For a woman to be referred for an abortion two doctors must confirm 'in good faith' that the gestation of the pregnancy is not greater than 24 weeks (counted from the first day of her last period) and that she meets one of several specified grounds. The exception to this is when the woman's life or health is in such danger that it constitutes a medical emergency. In this case a doctor can throw the rule book to wind, but any doctor doing so would have to be prepared to provide a sound justification for their actions, quite possibly in court. Outside the drama of medical emergencies, the grounds for abortions are as follows.

A. *The continuance of the pregnancy would involve risk to the life of the pregnant woman greater than if the pregnancy were terminated.*

In other words an abortion can be carried out if the woman's life is endangered by her pregnant state. This is very rarely ever the case, but an abortion might be judged to be life-saving if, for example, the woman was suffering from certain kinds of cancer, the growth of which are stimulated by pregnancy hormones. In cases such as this the 24 week time limit on abortion is waived. If the gestation of the pregnancy is such that child may be born alive every effort would be made to ensure that this is the case. However, a procedure where the intended outcome is a live birth is not classified as an abortion but an obstetric intervention.

There is an unresolved debate among doctors about whether the threat of suicide would be a legitimate reason for abortion under this clause. Some doctors agree that it would, others believe it would be more appropriate to detain the woman under the Mental Health Act!

B. *The termination is necessary to prevent grave permanent injury to the physical or mental health of the pregnant woman.*

When a woman suffers from a problem such as pre-eclampsia, a condition in which her blood pressure rises suddenly and threatens to cause kidney failure, a doctor may decide that an abortion is clinically in her best interest. As for Ground A the 24 week limit is waived, and if the gestation of the pregnancy is such that the child may be delivered alive every effort would be made to ensure that this would be the case.

C. *The continuance of the pregnancy would involve risk greater than if the pregnancy were terminated, of injury to the physical or mental health of the pregnant woman.*

The vast majority of early abortions, and nearly all abortions of unwanted pregnancies, are carried out under this provision. The clause is a controversial one as the terms 'risk' and 'health' are ambiguous.

Some doctors have argued that this clause in the act can allow very early abortion in *any* situation as, statistically, an abortion in early pregnancy is far less risky for the woman than carrying the baby to full term and undergoing labour.[6] Some doctors also argue that the term health should be interpreted broadly so as to include the states of anxiety and distress, two conditions experienced by every woman with an unplanned and unwanted pregnancy. Liberal doctors insist that the World Health Organization definition of 'health' as: 'a state of complete physical, mental and social well-being and not merely the absence of disease or infirmity' allows for this definition.

Interpreted liberally, this clause may allow a doctor to perform an abortion to save the woman from mental distress of a pregnancy that she does not wish to continue. However, doctors who are unsympathetic to a woman's situation may interpret it in such a way as to deny a woman an abortion unless she can demonstrate that continuing the pregnancy is going to reduce her to a state of clinical depression sufficient to require medical intervention.

The law specifically allows a doctor to take into consideration the pregnant woman's 'actual or reasonably foreseeable environment'. This means that factors such as the availability of support from a partner or family members, poverty, or living conditions can be considered.

D. *The continuance of the pregnancy would involve risk greater than if the pregnancy were terminated, of injury to the physical or mental health of any existing child(ren) of the family of the pregnant woman.*

This is the second most common ground by which women have abortions and is often used in the case of unplanned pregnancies. It may, on first consideration, be difficult to see how a child's physical health would be endangered by the birth of another, but perhaps a case can be made for this if another addition to the family would leave it in dire poverty or mean that either parent may not be able to provide the necessary care for the existing family.

E. *There is substantial risk that if the child were born it would suffer from such physical or mental abnormalities as to be seriously handicapped.*

There is no strict definition of either what constitutes a 'substantial risk' or a 'serious handicap' and both are matters of continuing controversy. However, there is general agreement that the circumstances in which these abortions are carried out are particularly tragic, as they are usually of much-wanted pregnancies.

A woman seeking to end an unplanned pregnancy in abortion is most likely to be referred under grounds (3) or (4).

The conscience clause

Doctors and other medical staff have the right to 'conscientiously object' to taking part in abortions unless medical treatment is necessary to save the life or prevent grave permanent injury to the woman. A doctor who conscientiously objects to abortion *should* refer the woman to a colleague who does not have such objections but this does not always happen. Sometimes, rather than explaining that he or she has a moral objection to abortion, a doctor will simply refuse to discuss the issue at all and in some cases he or she chooses to interpret the letter of the law very strictly and assert that the woman does not meet the legal requirements necessary for an abortion referral (see Gabrielle's story, below). A woman can, however, seek abortion advice or referral from *any* general practitioner, not just her own family doctor, and so if her own doctor objects she can in principle, immediately consult someone else. However, in some areas of the Midlands and the north-east of England the number of doctors who either conscientiously object or apply a strict interpretation to the law has rendered it virtually impossible for women to obtain abortions within National Health Service hospitals.

The contrast between these two accounts from students, both wishing to end an unwanted pregnancy by abortion shows how different interpretations of the law can be.

Gabrielle was a 20-year-old student at Manchester University when she discovered she was pregnant.

'I was at the doctor's surgery first thing in the morning and I explained to him that I was pregnant and I needed an abortion. He asked me why, and I explained that I simply did not want a child. It seemed straightforward to me. I didn't want to be pregnant and I didn't want a baby. Even the thought of it was awful. It wasn't that I didn't love my boyfriend. I did and we'd talked about getting married when we graduated and had jobs and all that. A baby would be the end of everything. They didn't even have a nursery at the University. I would have had to have given up my course, my parents would have killed me, this was the biggest disaster of my whole life.

'I blurted all this out and you could have cut the atmosphere with a knife. He was silent for about half a minute and then he said, "You can't just come in here and ask for an abortion like vitamin pills. You're young, intelligent, articulate, you're perfectly healthy, and you seem perfectly together. I can see no reason why you can't have your baby." Then he actually started to work out when it would be due and talk about future antenatal appointments. I couldn't believe it. I didn't think they could just say "No" like that.

Claire was 21 and in her final year at Reading University then she fell pregnant:

'I knew I was pregnant as soon as my period was late and I was so terrified. My parents are really strict Christians, they're the kind who even think sex before marriage is wrong. It would have killed them to know I was pregnant. I wasn't scared of having an abortion. If I had been more pregnant I might have felt differently about it but I was so early that I knew it was just a cluster of cells. The really strange thing was knowing that there's something growing in you and you don't want it to be there. It was very freaky.

'I saw a doctor at the family planning clinic. I told her that I was in trouble and she asked me lots of questions, things like, how did I know I was pregnant, what kind of contraception was I using, why did my boyfriend think, where was I living. She asked lots of things about me, not just about the pregnancy. For a moment I started getting worried because I didn't know why she needed to know all these things, especially because every now and again she'd make some notes. I think she sensed I was getting strung out because half way through the discussion she said that I wasn't to worry. There was no problem about arranging an abortion if I really felt that it was the best solution. She said it was clear that I wasn't in position to support a child financially and I'd probably got some growing up to do before I was mature enough for motherhood. She said that she wanted to make sure that I had considered other options, so that if I had the abortion I didn't regret it. That was a really great thing for her to say because once I knew it was going to be OK to have it, I did begin to think of other things to ask.

'I was given a leaflet which explained the different ways in which abortions were done and while I read it the doctor made an appointment for me to see someone at the hospital. She then suggested that I should come back and see her when this business was all over to discuss whether I should use a better type of birth control.'

The rights of men

Doctors quite often ask about the attitude of the man responsible for the pregnancy to the abortion. This is usually to establish whether the woman is under any psychological pressure from him either to get an abortion or to have the baby.

Neither a pregnant woman, nor a doctor from whom she seeks advice, is required by law to notify or consult the 'father' before the abortion is approved and he certainly has no right to veto a woman's decision. She, and she alone, has the right to decide whether or not to seek to have the pregnancy terminated in this way. If a doctor were to inform a woman's partner that she was intending to have an abortion, or even that she was pregnant, without her consent then the doctor would be in breach of his or her duty of confidentiality.

Northern Ireland

The 1967 Abortion Act does not apply to Northern Ireland, and the law there remains on paper the same as it was in the rest of the United Kingdom before the Act became law.

In Northern Ireland, abortion is, in principle, outlawed under the Offences Against the Person Act of 1861 which made it an offence for a woman to attempt to induce herself to miscarry, or for anyone else to assist in such an attempt unless the pregnancy is threatening her life. This absolute ban on abortion is tempered, as it was in England, by subsequent case law which allowed that there were circumstances when abortion might be legal. Notably, abortion might be legal when it was carried out by a member of the medical profession, acting in good faith to preserve the health of the woman.

The precise legal circumstances in which a woman can obtain a legal abortion in the province is unclear to the judiciary, the medical profession, and the public. Gynaecologists tend to make up their own rules as to when it is and is not appropriate to terminate a pregnancy. A survey carried out in 1994 by medical sociologist Colin Francome[7] found that some gynaecologists would carry out abortions only when there was evidence of fetal handicap, while others would terminate pregnancies only in cases of rape or incest. The Northern Ireland Standing Advisory Commission on Human Rights has, with the support of reproductive health care organizations, called for a review and clarification of the law.[8]

The tight restrictions on women obtaining legal abortion in Northern Ireland do not, however, prevent women from terminating un-planned pregnancies in this way. Each year around 2000 women with addresses in Northern Ireland have abortions in British clinics. These are joined by over 4000 women who cross from the Irish Republic, where the 'rights of the unborn child' are enshrined in the constitution. These figures, from both the North and the South of Ireland, are widely accepted to be a gross underestimate of the real extent of what has been described as 'abortion tourism'. Many women are thought to give false names and addresses out of fear that their secret abortion will be discovered. Some women still resort to amateur 'back street' abortion providers.

Gillian Douglas, a lecturer at the Cardiff Law School argues that the exodus of Irish women illustrates how ineffective the law is in preventing women from ending unwanted pregnancies. Faced with a restrictive law in one country, determined women will travel to another. Holland, for example, has a liberal abortion law, and Ireland prohibits abortions, yet proportionately just as many Irish women have abortions in Britain as Dutch women do in the Netherlands.[9]

How to get an abortion

This discussion of the law in the UK should allow you to understand the framework of the way the system works. We can now look at how women with unplanned, unwanted pregnancies can access the abortion service.

Step 1: confirm the pregnancy
Pregnancy tests, on sale over the counter in pharmacies are extremely accurate and confirm a pregnancy the day your period is due. How-ever, it is quite common to find that a positive pregnancy test is followed by a 'late period' within a matter of days. This does not mean that the test was falsely positive.

At least one-fifth of early pregnancies end in a spontaneous mis-carriage, and while a very early pregnancy test can detect a raised level of pregnancy hormones in your blood, it cannot show whether that pregnancy is likely to be sustained (see page 39 for more details).

Step 2: make an appointment with a doctor

You do not have to see your own doctor. If you suspect that your doctor may have objections to abortion, or even if you just think you may be more comfortable speaking to someone else, you can make an appointment with any other doctor—even one outside your practice. If there is a Brook Advisory Centre in your town, you can be confident of a sympathetic reception there. The medical staff at family planning clinics are also usually sympathetic to women seeking advice about abortion, but not all have a policy of referring women directly to hospital, and so you may find that after a discussion of the issues at the clinic you still have to find a GP to refer you to a hospital. In this case, however, the clinic may be able to suggest a sympathetic local GP.

If you are able to pay, you may prefer to bypass dealing with GPs and family planning doctors entirely and make an appointment at a charitable or private clinic. Two doctors will still need to approve the reason for the abortion, but the clinic will have doctors who can do this.

You may be worried that clinics outside the NHS provide an unsafe service. This is not the case: today's private clinics are carefully regulated and there is even an argument that they provide a better service as the clinics are specifically organized to provide a specialist service whereas NHS abortion referrals are usually slotted in amongst other gynaecology operations.

However, the prices charged by private clinics outside the charitable sector vary hugely, and you should always check that they are registered by the Department of Health.

Step 3: obtain the referral

As explained in some detail earlier in the chapter, you are not entitled to an abortion simply because you do not want to be pregnant. There is no clause in the abortion law that allows a doctor to refer you for an abortion because your pregnancy was unplanned or unwanted. He or she must complete a form indicating the legal grounds under which you are being referred and an offence is committed if your doctor fails to complete it, or if a case can be made that he or she has not acted in 'good faith'.

Before the appointment you may want to think about your life and your circumstances so that you can explain clearly why the pregnancy is a problem for you.

Step 4: get the appointment

This is where things can really slow down if you are trying to get an abortion within the NHS. Unfortunately, in most of England and

Wales abortions are provided as a part of the general gynaecology service which means they are slotted in amongst other gynaecology procedures. A hospital might, for example, plan for six abortions a week, and once these slots have been filled women are entered onto the list for the next week. This is a wholly inappropriate way in which to deal with abortion as the procedure by which it is carried out changes as the gestation of the pregnancy progresses. Abortions are very safe at any stage in pregnancy, but the later the abortion, the greater your risk of complications. Besides, once you have resolved to have the pregnancy terminated in this way you may be anxious to proceed quickly. In most areas of Scotland the situation is much better and the referral from a doctor to an appropriate hospital takes just a matter of days.

It is important to consider that some NHS hospitals will only carry out abortions after the twelfth week of pregnancy if there is a substantial risk of fetal abnormality or if there is a serious risk to your health which means that if there are long delays at any stage in the referral procedure you may find that an NHS abortion is no longer an option for you. Although there is a statutory duty for health authorities to meet the needs of their local community, it is down to them to decide which services they prioritize. There is no specific legal requirement for them to provide an abortion service. A woman's ease in obtaining an NHS abortion depends entirely on where she lives.

Once you have decided that you want an abortion, speed is of the essence. Make an appointment to see a doctor within a week of missing your period and when a doctor agrees to refer you, press them to make an appointment for you over the telephone there and then. If the hospital will only accept a referral by letter it may help to offer to take the letter along in person.

What happens during an abortion

Abortion has been practised as a means of fertility control in all communities throughout history. Anthropologists have found evidence of abortion practices in almost all societies, from the most primitive to the most sophisticated.[10] Potions, devices, and methods of massage to restore menstruation are documented as far back as ancient Egyptian, Greek, and Roman times.

Today the method of abortion used depends on the length of the pregnancy. This is calculated from the first day of the last menstrual period.

Abortion in early pregnancy

There are two methods of abortion available in the early weeks of pregnancy (before 12 weeks).

Vacuum aspiration or suction

This method is the most common method of abortion in Britain. It is routinely used when the pregnancy has a gestation of between eight and twelve weeks. Although the procedure can be carried out under a local anaesthetic (and is performed in this way in many other countries), most doctors in Britain prefer to use a general anaesthetic because the procedure is faster when the patient is unconscious.

The procedure is extremely simple. Once the woman has been anaesthetized the opening of the cervix is stretched from the normal 4 mm to the same number of millimetres as there are weeks in the pregnancy. Sometimes the cervix is softened with a pessary, which is placed in the vagina a few hours beforehand. A flexible plastic tube is then passed into the uterus and the contents are sucked out using an electric pump. This usually takes between 30 and 90 seconds.

After the abortion it is usual to experience some period-like bleeding and perhaps some stomach cramps for an hour or two. The slight bleeding may continue for five to ten days followed by a normal period after 28 to 35 days.

Vacuum aspiration abortions can be performed as day-cases without the need for an overnight stay. Most hospitals, however, either require the woman to stay the night before or the night after the operation.

Medical abortion

This is also known as RU 486, the 'abortion pill', Mifegyne or mifepristone. The abortion pill can be taken up to the end of the ninth week of pregnancy (63 days from the first day of the last period). The drug works by blocking the action of progesterone, the hormone which makes the lining of the uterus hold on to the fertilized egg. It is used in conjunction with a pessary containing a substance known as prostaglandin which makes the uterus cramp and speeds up the abortion. Medical abortion is not suitable for smokers over the age of 35.

Medical abortion involves three visits to the clinic or hospital, but an overnight stay is not usually required.

On the first visit the doctor gives the women tablets of mifepristone after which she is supposed to remain at the hospital for two hours in case she vomits before the drug has been absorbed into her system. The drug can only be given in an NHS hospital or in a clinic that has been licensed for abortion: it is not possible to obtain it from an ordinary GP.

After the administration of the tablets, the woman is free to leave the clinic and return home. But she *must* return for an appointment that will have been made for her in two days time. During the intervening period she may experience some period-like bleeding. In a few women, the tablets themselves may be sufficient to induce the abortion.

However, whether she bleeds or not, the woman will be required to return to hospital at an arranged time, where (except in the rare case where medical staff confirm that the abortion is complete) she will be admitted to a ward where she will stay for most of the day. A prostaglandin pessary is inserted into the woman's vagina, usually by a doctor or nurse, and shortly afterwards she will start to cramp and bleed.

The abortion usually takes place within eight hours of the insertion of the pessary. Most women experience strong crampy pains which are eased with analgesic pain killers. Some women also experience nausea, vomiting, or diarrhoea. A scan may be needed to determine whether the fetus and placenta have been passed in their entirety. At this stage in the pregnancy the fetus is still tiny, measuring just 1.5 cms in length and weighing only 1 gram.

Light bleeding continues for about 12 days after the abortion and the woman will be required to return for her third visit to the clinic seven days after the abortion to ensure that their are no retained products.

Although early medical abortion is routinely used in France it is not yet so common in Britain but it is offered by almost all the providers outside the NHS, and a growing number of NHS hospitals.

Choosing a method

There are advantages and disadvantages with both methods of early abortion, and what seems to be a disadvantage to one woman may seem to be an advantage to another. Here are some factors which you might want to consider.

Advantages of medical abortion

- If you have been referred for abortion very early in your pregnancy you may find it more acceptable to use the medical method than to wait until after the eighth week for vacuum aspiration.

- Some women describe the procedure as 'more like a natural miscarriage'.

- Some women find that being conscious throughout the procedure helps them to feel more in control of what is happening to their body.

- You may be able to have your partner or another companion with you throughout the abortion.

Advantages of vacuum aspiration abortion

- The procedure itself is very quick, and unless you are having a local anaesthetic, you will not experience the abortion itself.

- There are fewer visits to clinics involved and so this procedure may require less time off work or away from your family.

- There is no requirement for the clinic or hospital to inform your doctor—this may be important if you are trying to keep the abortion a secret. With early medical abortion the clinic or hospital must inform the woman's GP so that he or she is aware of her situation in the extremely rare event that any problems develop.

- There is less pain involved.

After twelve weeks

At 12 to 14 weeks the fetus becomes too bulky and firm to pass down the suction tube, so the method of abortion must be changed. Two main techniques are used.

Dilatation and evacuation

The woman is usually admitted to hospital the day before the abortion, and treatment is given to soften and open the cervix. The procedure is then carried out in an operating theatre under a light general anaesthetic. The cervix is dilated to about the same number of milli-metres as there are weeks in the pregnancy and then the fetus and placenta are crushed using special forceps and removed in fragments through the cervical opening. A suction tube may then be used to make sure there are no small pieces of tissue remaining in the uterus.

The procedure takes from five to 20 minutes. Recovery is swift and there is usually no post abortion pain.

Usually the woman can return home the same evening if the gestation was less than 16 weeks, but those with longer pregnancies may need to stay in hospital overnight. After 18 weeks this pro-cedure can still be used but it is more difficult. At this stage 'medical induction' would probably be used.

Medical induction

Medical induction is usual after 16 to 18 weeks and effectively involves inducing labour with prostaglandins.

Either a prostaglandin pessary is inserted into the vagina every three to six hours, or prostaglandin preparations can be injected into the uterus. An intravenous drip containing a drug that is used to stimulate labour at full term can also be used to make the process more efficient.

The woman will be fully conscious throughout the procedure and will have labour pains similar in length to those experienced when having a baby. Most women undergoing induction after 18 weeks are in labour for 11 hours, but between 5 and 15 per cent will take longer than 24 hours to expel the fetus. The fetus is expelled intact and is almost always dead. The woman may then have to be anaes-thetized to completely empty the uterus of all fragments of placenta and membrane.

Some hospitals use this method as early as 14 weeks. It has some advantages for the hospital because no surgical skill is necessary, and the procedure is considered to be more acceptable to many medical staff. However, the emotional stress of the abortion is far greater for the pregnant woman.

The change in the method of abortion, according to gestation shows how important it is for a woman seeking to end an unplanned pregnancy to obtain an early referral.

Preparing yourself

Before you are admitted to the hospital or clinic for the abortion it helps to find out as much as possible about what is going to happen. You may want to ask the following questions:

- How will the operation be performed?
- What kind of anaesthetic will be used?
- How long will I have to stay in hospital?
- What will I need to take with me to hospital?
- Will I be able to see a counsellor?
- Will my partner, a friend, or family member be able to be with me during the time that I am not in the operating theatre?
- Who will I contact if there are problems afterwards?

At the hospital or clinic the procedure will be similar to this description by BPAS director Ian Jones of what happens at one of his clinics when a woman is admitted for an early vacuum aspiration abortion.

'You will be allocated an appointment either first thing in the morning or at midday. If you have a morning appointment it is important not to eat or drink anything after 10 pm the night before. If you are booked in at lunch time, you can have a slice of toast and a drink at breakfast but nothing after. This is to make sure that you're not sick while you are under the anaesthetic.

'When you arrive at the clinic you will be booked in by the receptionist who will confirm all your personal details, including who will collect you after the operation. Day care patients must be collected by someone. If you are staying overnight you can go home alone the next day. The receptionist will also check what she should say if anyone telephones for you. You can leave a list of who you want to speak to, or take messages from. If anyone called who was not on the list the receptionist would deny all knowledge of you.

'You wait in reception until you're called up to the ward. When you get to the ward you have to undress and change into a gown—some clinics allow you to wear your own nightie. You have to remove all jewellery and make-up, even nail varnish. Jewellery is removed to prevent it from falling off in the theatre and make-up is removed so that the anaesthetist can see your true skin colour.

'You will be asked for a urine sample to make sure you are still pregnant, and a sample of blood to check your blood group and your rhesus status. All blood is either rhesus positive or rhesus negative (Rh+ or Rh−). When an Rh− women carries a Rh+ fetus, antibodies may build up in her blood which may cause problems in future Rh+ pregnancies. If you are one of the 15 per cent of women with Rh− blood you will be given an injection of anti-D immunoglobin to prevent this.

'When they are ready for you in surgery you are wheeled down on a trolley and the anaesthetic will be administered through a needle into the back of your hand.

'The next thing you will know is when you wake up in the recovery room. You may weep a little when you come round; this is a common side-effect of the anaesthetic. You will be wheeled back to the ward and you'll probably sleep for a couple of hours.'

The risks of abortion

Every medical treatment carries some risk and abortion is no exception, but the risks are *very* slight when the procedure is carried out by a competent medical practitioner.

Physical risks

It is statistically safer to have an abortion in early pregnancy than to carry the pregnancy to term. In general the risks increase with the gestation of the pregnancy, although vacuum aspiration abortions before eight weeks carry a slightly higher risk than those between eight and twelve weeks. This is because in the very early stage of the pregnancy the cervix is more difficult to dilate and the embryo and placenta are so small that they are easily missed. These problems do not arise with early medical abortion which can be carried out as soon as the pregnancy is confirmed.

Infections

Infections are the most common problems with early abortions. If a woman already has a sexually transmitted infection, such as chlamydia, present in her vagina, the abortion procedure may spread them into her uterus, turning a minor, symptomless infection into a more serious, painful one. Consequently, doctors are now advised to screen women for existing infections, such as chlamydia, before the abortion takes place.

Approximately one in 20 abortions will result in a mild infection and approximately one in 50 lead to an infection which requires hospital treatment. However, most infections that arise can be treated with a short course of antibiotics and many doctors prescribe women a prophylactic course of 'just-in-case' antibiotics after the operation to nip any developing infection in the bud.

Damage to the cervix or uterus

These are extremely rare in early pregnancy. The cervix is torn in about one abortion in a hundred. If this happens it can be repaired with a couple of stitches. Injuries to the uterine wall occur in fewer than one case for every 150 abortions.

Risk of infertility and future miscarriage

Published studies confirm that there is no link between abortion and infertility.[11] However, infertility can result from blockage or scarring of the fallopian tubes caused by post-abortion infections. There is also no evidence that women who have had early abortions are more prone to miscarriage in later pregnancies. There is a slight risk with later abortions where there is a greater risk of damage to the cervix. Smoking and deprived social circumstances are far more frequently associated with miscarriage than abortion.

Risk of death

Between 1981 and 1991, official statistics show a total of 13 deaths from abortion in England and Wales (ten in NHS and three in private clinics).[12] The NHS deaths were mainly before 1985, and since then the total annual deaths have been between zero and two per year. This means that the death rate from abortion has been about 0.7 per 100 000 abortions—the death rate from pregnancy as a whole, the maternal mortality rate, is about 10 times greater. These figures are comparable to those recently published in the United States of America where the death rate from legal abortion procedures between 1979 and 1985 was 0.6 per 100 000 procedures.[13]

Emotional risks

Precisely because abortion is a difficult decision for any woman, and because a significant section of society disapproves of abortion in principle, there are emotional risks attached to the operation that are absent from other medical procedures.

As discussed in chapter 2, the decision to have an abortion may be riddled with ambiguities. The woman might, perhaps, want to have a child at sometime in the future but not at this time in her life, or by the sexual partner by whom she has become pregnant. She herself may disapprove of abortion in principle, or her family or partner may disapprove of it. Few women go through the experience without experiencing feelings of sadness, regret, and remorse.

Sympathetic, non-directive counselling before the abortion can play an important role in allowing a woman to explore her feelings and doubts and make sure that she makes the right decision for her. Clinics and hospitals will provide the counselling before the abortion, and many provide the opportunity for further counselling after the procedure as well.

Society conspires to make women feel guilty about abortion. The very fact that the procedure is regulated by law sets it apart from other operations, making it clear that abortion should only be available in special circumstances when there are special reasons to excuse women from what would otherwise be their natural responsibility of motherhood. The disapproval of abortion by the church, and by some establishment figures and vocal campaigners adds to the pressure that a woman seeking an abortion may feel. Although between 35 and 40 per cent of all women in the population will have had an abortion by the time they reach the age of 45[14], the operation still carries a social stigma, and few women feel able to declare to the world that they have chosen to have a pregnancy terminated in this way. Often women find it easier either to claim that the pregnancy has spontaneously miscarried, or to tell no one of it at all.

The circumstances under which abortions are carried out in some hospitals can add to the emotional burden. Because women admitted to NHS hospitals for abortions are often treated as part of the general gynaecology intake, it is not uncommon for a woman admitted for an abortion to find herself in a bed alongside women being investigated for infertility or suffering from a miscarriage. This is distressing for all the women involved. There are also occasions where women may find themselves placed under the care of nursing staff who disapprove of abortion, perhaps not sufficiently to conscientiously object to being involved, but sufficient to make their views clear to the woman.

Under these circumstances it is not surprising that many women experience a sense of guilt or unease about their abortion.

A woman who goes ahead with the abortion—perhaps under pressure from her partner or because her family insists that she has an abortion—is more likely to suffer emotionally after the abortion. Women who have grown up among those who strongly disapprove of abortion are also more likely to suffer guilty feelings.

However, there is no medical evidence to suggest that abortion is responsible for deep long-lasting psychological trauma, or indeed even the onset of clinical depression, where it has not existed before the operation. A considerable amount of research on post-abortion trauma has been carried out, particularly in the United States where post-abortion problems are a subject of intense public debate. In 1989, after reviewing more than 250 studies Surgeon General C. Everett Koop concluded that the emotional problems resulting from abortion are 'minuscule from a public health perspective.'[15]

When American psychiatrist Dr Paul K. B. Dagg reviewed 225 published medical papers on the psychological aspects of abortion he concluded that:

> 'Immediately after the abortion symptoms of distress and dysphoria [sadness] do occur in many women. However, these symptoms seem to be continuous of symptoms present before the abortion and more a result of circumstances leading to the abortion than a result of the procedure itself. Indeed many studies report significant positive feelings after the abortion. When the women are studied over the course of the episode, the dysphoria is found to be on the wane after the abortion. Longer-term studies, over months and years, show similar trends; the majority of women express positive attitudes to the abortion and only a small minority express any degree of regrets. Similarly, negative feelings before the abortion disappear, with normalisation of various scores.[16]

In short: most women feel sad at the time but have no long term depression or anxiety after abortion.

A woman can experience remorse, sadness, and regret, whilst still feeling that she has made the right decision. Her grief may be that it was necessary to make that decision at all. She may even need time to mourn for what might have been had the circumstances in her life been different and allowed her to make other decisions about her pregnancy.

The moral maze

There are dozens, perhaps hundreds, of books on medical ethics which discuss the rights and wrongs of abortion in the abstract. But for each individual woman with an unplanned pregnancy the issue of whether an abortion is morally right or wrong is a question that ultimately she must answer for herself. Only she knows what the consequences of continuing the pregnancy will mean and only she knows whether she would cope better if she ended it.

The moral rights and wrongs of abortion are often discussed as though the issue is a philosophical debate, but for a woman with an unplanned pregnancy the discussion is extremely practical. The decisions that she takes now will influence her for the rest of her life.

During her pregnancy a woman is not simply an incubator who lives in a state of suspended animation until the baby pops out ready to be accepted into her life or adopted by someone else. Pregnancy brings about many changes to every aspect of a woman's life, many of which she may find intolerable. Thousands of women who are opposed to the idea of abortion 'in principle' find it the only practical solution to their own unplanned, unwanted pregnancy.

It is beyond the scope of this book to discuss the rights and wrongs of legal abortion. The fact that it *is* legal enables it to be an option for many tens of thousands of women every year. However, given that abortion is perceived to be a controversial topic the final section of this chapter will look at the most well-known arguments voiced by those who oppose and support women's right to abortion.

The arguments against legal abortion

There are those who sincerely believe that the very existence of legal abortion is an abomination against humanity. A minority, but a significant minority, none the less, believe that abortion is an act of moral depravity equivalent to murder—perhaps worse, as the fetus is so helpless and innocent.

Two of the most common arguments against abortion are the following.

Life begins at conception

Many of those who object to abortion base their moral stance on the principle that human life begins at conception and that from that moment the status of a 'human being' should be accorded. From that moment, to those who accept this principle, a human being with rights essentially the same as those belonging to ordinary adults is present. It follows from this that any deliberate act which results in the destruction of the embryo or fetus is tantamount to murder. The fetus, often referred to as an 'unborn' or 'preborn' baby is accorded the 'right to life'.

This attitude is held by the Catholic church and is justified in the 1974 *Declaration on Procured Abortion* which reads:

'In reality respect for human life is called for from the time that the process of generation begins. From the time that the ovum is fertilised, a life is begun which is neither that of the father nor that of the mother; it is the life of a new human being with his own growth. It would never be made human if he were not human already.'

This view has been endorsed by successive popes, and accepted by some outside the Catholic tradition.

Those who support legal abortion argue that uncompromising support for the sanctity of life does not seem to be consistently sustained even by many people with strong religious beliefs, who often accept that there are times, as in war, when it is legitimate to sacrifice life. They suggest that it also fails to take into consideration the fact that God, or nature, does not seem to accord much respect to the early pregnancy—given that at least 20 per cent end in spontaneous miscarriage and that, as there is no provision to bury miscarried fetuses in holy ground, or indeed conduct funerals for them, it is somewhat inconsistent to accord them full human rights in respect of the discussion on abortion.

Another argument is that it is absurd to suppose that an embryo with no sense of self-awareness should be accorded the same status as an adult person and that there is a difference between the status of 'potential person' (which the embryo or fetus is accorded) and an 'actual person'.

Moral responsibility

Many who oppose abortion on principle, or who believe it should only be made available in the most tightly restricted circumstances, believe that fundamental to sexuality is the issue of responsibility. If a woman becomes pregnant it is seen as her moral responsibility to endure the consequences of her actions and have the child. This view is frequently expressed by those who would identify themselves as 'moral conservatives' and who believe that the liberalization of abortion laws has contributed to a decline in moral/sexual standards.

This argument is countered by those who insist that it is acceptable to regard sex as a recreational activity, and that even those who practise it responsibly are at risk of pregnancies which they do not want, and can perhaps ill-afford. It is argued that to bring an unwanted child into the world is problematic for the child as well as for the parents. There is, in any case, no evidence that countries in which abortion is outlawed have higher moral/sexual standards than those in which it is easily available.

The arguments for legal abortion

Of course, just as some people believe passionately that abortion should be criminalized, there are those who believe with equal conviction that the law should be liberalized and that abortion should be available as a woman's right.

These 'pro-choice' arguments are in general based on the principle that a woman should be able to make choices about her reproductive future, and that no woman should be forced to bear a child that she does not want.

Two common arguments for legal abortion are the following.

Women's equality and individual choice

Many who support the principle of women's right to abortion believe it to be an essential component of women's autonomy and independence. They argue that they are pro-choice rather than pro-abortion and believe no one should have the right to override a woman's choices about her own body and fertility. It is sometimes argued that given the rate of unplanned pregnancy the denial of access to abortion places women on an unequal footing with men.

It is also argued that decisions about abortion can only be made by the individual woman as only she knows and understands the problems that continuing the pregnancy will cause.

Those who oppose legal abortion believe that abortion can no more be seen as an issue of individual moral conscience than can, say, the struggle against genocide or slavery. If a wrong is being done then it is the responsibility of society to correct it. Thus they argue that even if a woman wishes to terminate her pregnancy it is appropriate for others to veto that choice. It is also argued that abortion, rather than assisting women to equality, has enabled men to take advantage of them sexually without having to worry about the consequences of fatherhood. This is countered by the argument that a woman may enjoy recreational sex as much as a man and may be just as anxious, if not more so, to escape parenthood as a consequence.

The unequal status of the woman and the fetus

Most people who condone abortion believe that the rights of the fetus are not equal to those of the women. The fetus is often accorded some moral status—but as a *potential* human life rather than a human being in its own right. A fetus might be alive (in the sense that it is not dead) and human (in the sense that it is not, say, a gerbil) but it does not have the qualities of human life that we specifically respect. It does not know that it is alive, it is not even conscious. Furthermore, it is argued that it is not possible for a fetus to exercise any supposed rights, except through the mother, and that the fetus cannot be accorded rights without compromising the rights of the woman.

This is countered by the argument that an individual life begins at conception, and that lack of consciousness does not detract from the fact that life, biologically exists. Those who oppose abortion insist that the right of a woman to live as she please is inequitable to the right of the unborn child to live, and a woman has no right to sacrifice a life to maintain her life-style.

In conclusion

The arguments for and against abortion have raged for centuries and will continue to be debated—amongst philosophers, ethicists, and politicians. For a woman, however, the decision to continue or end her pregnancy is usually made more on the basis of practical considerations than on moral principles. This is not because women care less about morals or ethics but because sometimes the circumstances in which we live force us to compromise our beliefs and choose between a variety of options, all of which are distressing. A woman with an unwanted pregnancy faces a range of choices none of which she *wishes* to make. An American pro-choice activist explains the decision like this: 'A woman doesn't want an abortion in the way that she wants a holiday, she wants it as an animal in a trap wants to gnaw off its foot to escape.'

Those who counsel women with unwanted pregnancies find that many women who object to abortion in principle nevertheless choose it as a solution to their own problem because they feel it to be the 'lesser evil' of the options available. The fact that they have themselves had an abortion does not necessarily alter their view that it is 'wrong'.

Evidence from around the world suggests that even when women live in societies in which abortion is forbidden they will use whatever means necessary to procure one. In the UK, even before the Abortion Act came into force in 1968, it was estimated that between 50 000 and 250 000 women underwent illegal abortions each year. Today in Brazil, women suffering from failed amateur abortions fill 30 per cent of the beds in the women's wards of Rio de Janeiro hospitals. In Europe, many women travel, often at great cost, from countries where abortion is tightly restricted to those with more permissive laws. Women from Germany, which has restrictive laws, travel to the Netherlands. In the early 1980s before abortion was legalized in Spain, as many as 20 000 Spanish women travelled to Britain for abortions every year. As we have already discussed, more than 6000 women still cross the Irish Sea to that end.

In Britain, abortion is an episode in very many women's lives. There should be no cause for shame, or apology, and indeed, there is none.

Before we move on to look at the alternative choices facing women with unplanned pregnancies, here are the accounts of four very different women who chose to have abortions.

Mary's story

Mary is 25 and married with a young son. She is Irish although she has lived in Liverpool since she was six. She is the only daughter of staunchly Catholic parents.

'I felt very ashamed about it, and I still do feel ashamed. Nobody knows except my husband.

'We've always been careful about birth control. We're quite religious, but not so religious that we don't use birth control. And we were extra careful because we do believe abortion is a sin. In my heart I do believe it is wrong, but sometimes I think you have to do something that's wrong to stop something even more wrong.

'I don't know how I got pregnant, we always used condoms and neither of us knew what went wrong, but I knew I was in the family way as soon as I didn't 'come on' when I should have. Believe me, to have had that baby would have been as big a sin as I could have made. Sean [her husband] was on the sick. He's a builder and he had hurt his back, and my little one had been in hospital with a bad chest. I was running around like a maniac looking after the both of them.

'I want another child, I love children but this was the worst time. Sean and I discussed it, we both cried over it. I was so scared. I had never known of a married woman having an abortion. I thought they would think so badly of me at the clinic, and that they might say there was no reason. After all it's different when you're 15, or you've been raped or something. I was also really scared that the nurses would think I was sinning. I don't know why I worried more about the nurses than the doctors, but I did.

'We had saved a little money, and I went to a clinic in Liverpool. I got the address by calling somewhere in London—I couldn't face my doctor to ask him. I hated having to pay—it made me feel so ashamed, really cheap and as though it was something I shouldn't really be doing. It was as though I had to bribe someone. But when I met the other women who were having abortions it made me feel better. They were just normal women. Every time I think of abortion now I think of ordinary women, and ordinary women's problems.'

Susie's story

Susie is a 36-year-old personnel manager. She is divorced and had an abortion nine years ago.

'At the time I had no regrets about the operation. It seemed the most sensible thing to do. I was too immature to be a mother. I really was very young for my age. Looking back I think I was too young to be married. I never really 'discussed' it with my husband—I think I just sort of 'told' him—which was typical of our relationship. That's why we split up, we never really talked about anything.

'Now I do regret it. I feel I might have missed my one chance to have a child. I'm not in a relationship at the moment and I know that my biological clock is ticking away. The first grey hairs are showing through and all that. It suddenly occurred to me that I might go all through my life and never know what it's like to give birth and breast feed—yet I could have done it if I had wanted to then. It's all very complicated.

'It's amazing how your feelings change over the years. Ten years ago I thought women who wanted babies were certifiable—totally mad. Now I always find I pay particular attention to children who are nine or ten, about the age that mine would have been. I sometimes have imaginary conversations with my daughter. Perhaps I'm the one who's going mad!

'Looking back, though it is hard to say, if I put myself in the position I was then, I wonder whether I would make the same decision. If I hadn't made that decision, who knows what would have happened. I wouldn't be the same person I am now, so maybe I'd feel different about it. It's too complicated to even think about.'

Beccy's story

Beccy is a 24-year-old hotel receptionist. She is single with no children. She had an abortion a year ago using the abortion pill.

'I did not for one minute consider anything other than an abortion. I suppose I was lucky because my friends are all pro-choice, and we grew up believing in women's rights to this kind of thing. I had often wondered how I would feel if it were me that was pregnant, but I just felt angry and cheated. I knew that I had taken a risk but then so do thousands of other people and they don't get caught. There was no question of having the baby. I didn't even think of it as a baby, just a huge great problem.

'I had read about the abortion pill in a magazine article, and it seemed like a good way to have it done. I liked the idea of not having to have a general anaesthetic. I hated the idea of doctors poking around and me not knowing what they were doing. The abortion pill seemed more natural.

'I had the abortion at a clinic in south London. It was more of a performance than I expected. First I had to go and see one doctor there, then I had to see someone who wasn't a doctor but explained what would happen and how I might feel. Then I had another appointment where I saw a second doctor and I had the tablets.

'I was nearly sick after I'd taken them, but I think it was because I felt sick nearly all the time with the pregnancy. People forget about that—how pregnancy makes you feel, it's terrible. After the tablets I was a bit nervous, I never had any second thoughts about the abortion, but I was nervous about what would happen when I started bleeding. I kept going to the bathroom every half hour to see if anything was happening but I didn't start bleeding until the day I was due to go back to the clinic. I went to the toilet and there was blood—just like my period was starting. I was so pleased I wanted to dance. When you're pregnant and you don't want to be you want a period more than anything else in the world.

'There were four of us at the clinic which was great because we all got on really well—I suppose we were in the same boat. We weren't put into beds, which was a bit of a surprise. The doctor put the pessary in. I was hoping I wouldn't have to have one as I was bleeding quite a lot.

'I started cramping quite soon after, which was really painful—much worse than period pain. One of the other girls was so bad she needed an injection, but the rest of us could manage with painkillers. I wasn't aware of exactly when the abortion took place because I was passing lots of quite big clots of blood.

'Afterwards a nurse talked to me about contraception, and about how important it was for me to go back for a check up, she said to call at any time if I was worried or I wanted to talk about things. That was the only thing I hated about it—everybody seemed to be walking on eggshells, as if I ought be guilty and upset. As it was it started to make me feel guilty because before I didn't feel guilty. But in the end, what kind of life would a child have with me, now.

'I can honestly say that the only time I felt bad was when a friend told me she was starting infertility treatment. Life is so unfair.'

Judith's story

Judith is a 40-year-old teacher. She is married with two children aged eight and twelve. She had an abortion two years ago.

'It was a really difficult decision, but neither my husband nor I really wanted another child. We felt the family was complete and we were relieved that the two boys were out of the baby stage.

'I knew I was pregnant right away because I recognized all the feelings. Peter [her husband] and I talked about it. He said it had to be my decision and he would support me whatever I decided, which was nice, but at the same time it threw all the responsibility onto me.

'We decided I would have an abortion because neither of us felt we could cope emotionally with looking after a young baby. When I hear people argue that women should give children up for adoption rather than have abortions it makes me angry. I could never have given a child away after I had carried it and given birth to it. I couldn't cope with knowing my child was out there somewhere.

'We decided to pay for the abortion—just to get it done as quickly as possible. I knew that the longer I was pregnant the more doubts I would have. We didn't tell anyone. My mother looked after the children for the two days I was away. I told her that I had to go into hospital for a couple of days for some investigations because my periods had been all over the place. She may have suspected what was going on, but she has never asked about it.

'I don't think about it all that much—only occasionally I wonder if it would have been a girl.

References

1. Office of Population Censuses and Surveys, Abortion Statistics 1993, Series AB no. 18. HMSO, London.
2. Smith, T. (1993). Influence of socioeconomic factors on attaining targets for reducing teenage pregnancies. *British Medical Journal*, **307**, 1233–35.
3. Paintin, D. (1994). Why abortion services are necessary. In D. Paintin (ed.). *Abortion services in England and Wales*, p. 19. BCT, London.
4. Royal College of Obstetricians and Gynaecologists (1991). *Report of the RCOG working party on unplanned pregnancy*, p. 10. RCOG, London.
5. Office of Population Censuses and Surveys, Abortion Statistics 1993, Series AB, no. 18. HMSO, London.

6. For a detailed discussion of this point see: Mason, J.K. (1990). *Medico-legal aspects of reproduction and parenthood*, pp. 106–7, Sweet and Maxwell, London.
   Douglas, G. (1991). *Law, fertility and reproduction*, pp. 89–92. Sweet and Maxwell, London.
7. Francome, C. (1994). Gynaecologists and abortion in Northern Ireland. *Journal of Biosocial Science*, **25**, 389–94.
8. See A. Furedi (ed.) (1995). *Human rights and reproductive choice: the abortion law in Northern Ireland*. Family Planning Association Northern Ireland, Belfast.
9. Ketting, E. and van Praag, P. (1986). The marginal relevance of legislation relating to induced abortion. In J. Lovenduski and J. Outshourn (eds) *The new politics of abortion*, pp. 154–69. Sage, London.
10. Devereux, G. (1976). *A study of abortion in primitive societies*. International Universities Press, New York, NY.
11. Frank, P. *et al.* (1993). The effect of induced abortion on subsequent fertility. *British Journal of Obstetrics and Gynaecology*, **100**, 575–80.
12. Office of Population Censuses and Surveys, Abortion Statistics 1993, Series AB no. 18. HMSO, London.
13. Council on Scientific Affairs (1992). Induced termination of pregnancy before and after Roe v. Wade: trends in the mortality and morbidity of women. *Journal of the American Medical Association*, **268**, 3231–39.
14. Paintin, D. (1994). Why abortion services are necessary. In D. Paintin (ed.): *Abortion services in England and Wales*, p. 17. BCT, London.
15. Testimony of Surgeon General to House of Representatives, Hearings before the House of Representatives and Inter-Governmental Relations Sub Committee of the Committee on Government Operations and House of Representatives, 101st Congress, 1st Session (1989). Testimony of C. Everett Coop.
16. Dagg, P.K.B. (1991). The psychological sequelae of therapeutic abortion—denied and completed. *American Journal of Psychiatry*, **148**, 578–85.

5

Considering adoption

Adoption is the least common solution to unplanned pregnancy nowadays, probably because it involves all the stresses of pregnancy and labour but with none of the joys of motherhood after the birth. The claim that today adoption is seen as the least socially acceptable solution to unplanned pregnancy is probably true. A study of the attitudes of single mothers conducted in the late 1970s showed that of 36 unmarried, pregnant young women, only one said she would choose adoption, while 18 dismissed adoption immediately as intolerable. Abortion, single parenting, or getting married were, by far, the preferred choices.[1] Today, it is probably even less acceptable to most women. In 1991 just 1115 babies under one year old were adopted. When this figure is compared to the 12 641 adoption orders granted in respect of babies under one year old in 1968, it is clear how attitudes to adoption have altered.

Today, the main purpose of adoption seems to have changed. While in a relatively small number of cases it still has its traditional function of providing a home for a new baby that a mother is unable to raise, adoption is increasingly used as a way of removing children from situations that social services agencies have defined as being 'at risk'—if, for example, they believe the child is being, or will be, abused. This means that, today, more adoption orders involve older children than babies. In 1968, more than three-quarters of adoption orders (76 per cent) involved babies under 12 months old; by 1984 the proportion of orders involving babies under one year was less than half (46 per cent). The new role of adoption is, unfortunately, a separate issue and beyond the scope of this book. This chapter concentrates on adoption only as a possible solution to an unplanned pregnancy.

There are two main reasons why adoption is a relatively uncommon solution to the problem of unplanned pregnancy.

The availability of abortion

For many women, abortion was, and still is, the 'lesser evil' of the options because the fact of pregnancy can be concealed. No one need ever know it happened, not even the man responsible, if the woman confides in no one.

The acceptability of single motherhood

It is now regarded as socially acceptable for a woman to become pregnant before she marries, even before she is in a stable relationship. Thus more women feel they are able to raise a child which in a different, more conservative society they may have felt under pressure to give up.

Studies suggest that the adoption option was never a *favoured* choice by women, it was rather an 'only option'—the sole alternative to disgrace of a 'shot-gun wedding'. In a study of the sexual behaviour and attitudes of young people in the early 1960s, when the girls were asked what they would do in the event of an unplanned pregnancy, all said they would wish to keep the child[2], but in practice adoption was usually preferable to the social death of single motherhood.

A small in-depth study of 49 women who relinquished a child for adoption at this time[3] found that the stigma of unmarried motherhood, particularly in the form of negative reaction from family and friends was their main reason for going through with the procedure.

The authors record a powerful list of comments from the women interviewed:

'My parents would not consider helping me to keep her. They could have but the stigma was too much for them at that time.'

'I never felt anything to be ashamed of but they did.'

'They were so ashamed that they just totally rejected me; my mother would actually pass me in the street without a word.'

'I had to leave my home, my job, my friends because I was so ashamed.'

'Horror—everything must be hidden from friends and neighbours. The one or two who knew would use a special signal on the front door so that I did not have to go and hide in my room.'

'Only my mother knew. She made me pack my bags as soon as I told her and it was three years before we spoke again. She was absolutely terrified of the scandal. She has never referred to the incident since that time and nor have I.'

'My father was furious. There were no visits, no contact in hospital, no discussions about the baby. It was as though the whole thing never happened.'

Even when families showed sympathy and understanding there was seldom any serious consideration given to keeping the baby.

Today, attitudes towards births outside marriage and single motherhood have changed beyond recognition. Although single women with babies do still attract disparaging comments, there is now less stigma attached to single motherhood than at any time in modern history. Rising divorce rates have contributed to a situation where a third of families are headed by just one parent and the more liberal attitude to sex means that a lone woman with a child is no longer seen as shameless. This means that many women who might in the past have felt unable to raise a child alone now have no qualms whatsoever about embarking on that road.

Because the decision to relinquish a baby for adoption is relatively uncommon, it is often difficult for women with unplanned pregnancies to obtain information on what the adoption procedure involves from their point of view. Most books on adoption are written for the far greater number of people who wish to adopt, or have been adopted. The authors of *Half a Million Women*[4], one of the few books which discusses the experience of women who have given up their children, point out that society does not even have an adequate name for such women, although our vocabulary is rich in labels. The term 'birth mother' is usually used, but this is an unsatisfactory label because it applies to any mother—not just those going into the adoption process.

Although adoption is a relatively unpopular choice for women today, it is an important choice nevertheless. Many women, especially those with strongly held religious convictions feel abortion to be unacceptable, and yet know they would be unable practically to rear their child, even if that is what ideally they would wish to do. For them adoption may still seem to be the *only* option.

Other women, not all of them religious, may gain a great deal of satisfaction from their involvement in what is sometimes described as a 'double-gift relationship': the gift of life to a child, and the gift of a child to a family who long for one. For some women this may be a way for them to turn the bad situation of an unintended pregnancy into a fortuitous one. It may even seem to be a way of atoning for the mistakes of the past.

There are as many reasons why women have their children adopted as there are children who have been adopted. For some women it is the only choice they feel able to make, others may find themselves going down this road by default if, for example, they have, for whatever reason, been unable to arrange an abortion sufficiently early in pregnancy.

This chapter highlights some of the issues that need to be considered.

What is adoption

Adoption is a way for the 'birth' parents to cut legal ties with their child and to allow him or her to be provided with new legal parents. The process effectively ends the legal relationship between the child and the birth parents and establishes a new one with adoptive parents. Once an adoption order has been granted it is final and cannot be revoked.

When a woman is unsure whether she wants to have the child adopted it may be appropriate for her to consider having the child placed with foster parents. Fostering is an arrangement whereby the child becomes a member of another family for a temporary period. This arrangement can last for week,s months, or occasionally years and it can provide a useful breathing space to allow a woman or a couple to sort out their life.

The law and how it works

Adoption procedure is strictly regulated by law. The Adoption Act, which became law in 1976 was passed to codify all the various rules and regulations which related to the procedure. The Act, which runs to 56 pages, covers every facet of adoption in fine detail, including the following aspects.

Who can arrange adoptions?

Every local authority must, by law, run a service designed to meet the needs of all involved: the birth parents, the adoptive parents, and the child. This should include temporary housing arrangements for pregnant women intending to give up their child. The local authority must also ensure that everyone involved has access to counselling.

In practice, adoptions are arranged by the Social Services Department (or Social Work Department in Scotland) of the local authority and by specially approved voluntary agencies. All these organizations have specially trained social workers who are able to discuss the issues involved. In addition, most hospitals employ social workers who work with maternity clinics.

It is not possible for an individual or couple to make their own arrangements unless the child is to be adopted by a very close family member. However, it is possible for the birth parents to specify some things about the kind of parents they would like. By law, the adoption agency must take account of their wishes with regard to the religious upbringing of the child; in practice they also consider other factors. Wherever possible agencies try to place children with adoptive parents who are of the same ethnic and cultural origin as the birth parents.

Who can adopt

Those who wish to adopt are subject to quite careful scrutiny by the adoption agencies. There are no regulations to prevent single people from adopting, and in fact the law specifically provides for this, but the adoption agency must be certain that they will be able to cope with raising a child.

The welfare of the child

For the agencies involved in adoption, the welfare of the child is paramount. The law specifically states that the first responsibility of any adoption agency is to 'safeguard and promote the welfare of the child throughout his childhood' (Adoption Act 1976, part I, section 6). This means that throughout the process the adoption agency has the right to override the wishes of both the birth parents and the adoptive parents, if they feel that it is in the interests of the child to do so.

Normally, a birth mother can change her mind and have the child returned to her at any time before the adoption is finalized, but this is not always the case. For example the wishes of the birth parents can be set aside if they are thought to be withholding agreement 'unreasonably', have 'persistently failed without reasonable cause to discharge parental duties in relation to the child' or have 'abandoned', 'neglected' or 'persistently ill treated' the child.

Birth records

A National Adopted Children Register is maintained by the Registrar General and contains birth records of adopted children. These are not generally available to the public, but details from the register may be obtained by adopted children themselves once they have reached adulthood. The details available are those on the birth certificate, which include the name of the birth mother and her address at the time the child was born. It may have her maiden name, if she was married, and it may also contain the name, address, and occupation of the birth father. Through these details it has been possible for some adopted children, often using considerable detective skills, to trace their birth parents. The Children Act, passed in 1989, allowed for the setting up of an Adoption Contact Register. This was established in the recognition that many adopted children wish to know more than the basic information on the birth certificate and that many birth parents were happy for their details to be known and to provide a more systematic way for adopted children and birth parents to make contact (see pp. 111–13).

Making the decision

The adoption process has been transformed over the years. Until the 1970s, it was the vogue for young, unmarried, pregnant women to be sent off to an institution six weeks before the birth of the child. She would emerge approximately six weeks after the birth, when the child would be placed for adoption. The mother would be expected to return to her previous circumstances and resume her life as though nothing had happened.

Today most women remain at home until they are admitted for delivery and into appropriate maternity care in much the same way as any other pregnant women. The Life Care and Housing Trust runs a network of 'Life Houses' where accommodation can be found for women whose circumstances would otherwise lead them to have abortions, and local authorities may be able to provide some practical assistance to young women who are unable, for whatever reason, to remain at home until the child is born and relinquished.

The way in which pregnant women intending to relinquish their children are treated in the 1990s carries different pressures to those on women a couple of decades ago. A study of unmarried parents in the late 1960s described the terrible situation faced by a birth mother intending to relinquish her baby: society blames her shuffling off her responsibilities, while she undergoes the pangs of real bereavement without the sympathy and understanding that would have been hers had the baby died. She is left with the memory of a demanding and helpless infant, and a constant unfulfilled desire to know how he is getting on.[5]

Today, this should no longer be the case. The emotional needs of birth mothers are recognized and are taken account of. Counselling and emotional support are available and, while women can never be protected from insensitive remarks and even perhaps the occasional deliberately cruel comment, everything is done by the professional agencies involved to support the birth mother through the experience.

One of the most difficult aspects of the adoption option is that it involves living with uncertainty for a long time. Many women find that they have doubts as to whether they will be able to go through with it until the adoption order is granted.

The decision is usually a consequence of a careful weighing up of the conflicting interests. These are often the interests of others (which often manifests itself in the form of pressure from parents or partner), the interests of the future child, and self-interest.

Your decision

Before you decide whether adoption is the right option for *you*, you may want to consider these questions.

- What does the father want?
- How will I cope with the practical aspects of pregnancy; for example, can I take maternity leave from my job?
- How will my family and friends react, and what support will they give me?
- How might I feel as the birth gets nearer?
- Will I want to explain to people that I intend to have the child adopted?
- How will I feel about the involvement of social workers?
- How much will I want to know about the adoptive parents?
- What kind of family would I like my child to have?
- How certain am I that I want to have the baby adopted rather than fostered?
- How will I feel knowing that I have a child who doesn't know me?
- How might the decision affect my future relationships?

The interests of others

Pressure from family, particularly parents, is often a significant factor in the decision, especially with younger women who may feel completely powerless to resist it. This is particularly the case if the young woman is living at home with no independent income. The situation that 15-year-old Sandy found herself in is typical of many teenagers with unplanned pregnancies.

'If I had found out earlier that I was pregnant I would probably have had an abortion. As it was I was four months gone by the time I knew and it was another month before I got to tell mum. My monthlies were all over the place anyway, and I just kept hoping it would start.

'In some ways I would have liked to have kept the baby but everybody made it clear from the start that there was no chance of that. My mum said that she had spent just as much time looking after babies as she was prepared to, and she wasn't having another one in the house. You can understand why. We've only got a small place, and I suppose she's right that she would have been saddled with a lot of the work.

She went mental when I said I wanted to keep him. She went on and on about how I couldn't be trusted to feed the cat, so how was I going to look after a kid.

'But I did want him. I went to find out about one of those hostels run by the Catholics. They said I could go there if my mum threw me out. But it's not really on is it. What happens when you have to leave? You're on your own

'It was worst at the hospital. Although, because I look young, people were very nice about it. I think a lot were quite relieved when I said he was being adopted because they couldn't handle thinking that I was going to bring him up myself. My mum took charge of everything, all the arrangements.

'I never feel guilty about giving him away. In some ways I'm quite proud. I know girls who've had abortions, but I think even if I never do anything else, at least I brought a life into the world.'

Pressure from the partner is another major consideration. A woman who strongly wishes to keep her child may feel unable to do so if she feels (or knows!) that her partner will withdraw his support, or perhaps end the relationship. If her partner has strong anti-abortion beliefs, adoption may be chosen by a woman who would otherwise have had an abortion.

The interests of the child

Often the decision to relinquish the child for adoption is made because it is thought to be in the child's best interests, despite the fact that the birth mother would really like to keep it. Penny, who became pregnant from a 'one-night stand' when she was unemployed and with no means of support except state benefit, never accuses her social worker of manipulating her, but it is hard not to suspect that if she had encountered a more encouraging attitude her decision about her baby may have been different.

'It broke my heart to give Patrick away. I still dream about him and sometimes I wake up and I can smell that sweet baby smell. But what could I give him? Looking back I can see that the social worker influenced me a lot about the adoption. We'd have these conversations which would start off about how I was going to handle things and end up talking about all the people with all the money in the world who could have a family. I would always feel so twisted up. Every time there was anything on the news about 'unfit mothers' I'd go mental because I knew they meant women like me. There were times when I would be really bolshie about it, but then as the birth got closer I got scared. And I could see they were really all right. I felt I'd messed up my life and I didn't have the right to mess up any one else's.'

Sociological studies of adoption[6] note that discussions between 'professional carers' and single women, particularly those from economically disadvantaged backgrounds, frequently place the birth mother with a pernicious choice: if you really love the baby you will give her up to someone who can give her a better life; if you keep the child you are being selfish and do not love her enough.

Although 20-year-old Stephanie, a student, had come to an agreement with her boyfriend that they would have the child and try to settle down as a family, she was told by her midwife, 'if you're not sufficiently responsible to use contraception, what makes you think you are up to rearing a child.' Having been made to feel like a selfish child herself, she became convinced that adoption probably was for the best.

Self-interest

Often women feel a need to deny their own self-interest in the matter, perhaps as a way of displacing responsibility for the decision onto other people. But sometimes it is important for a woman to face up to the fact that adoption may be the best decision she can make for herself.

Helen gave up her baby for adoption when she was 22 and sees it as a 'positive, important choice'.

'I'm not ashamed of it—in some ways I'm rather proud of myself for going through with it. Of course I regret getting pregnant, it was stupid and wrong, but I feel I've atoned for that by my actions since. My baby has gone to a family where he'll be loved and cherished and I'm sure that's for the best for us both. If I had kept him I wouldn't have been able to finish my degree, and I think it would have ruined my chances of finding the kind of man I want to settle down with. Whatever people say, men do not want to take on the responsibility of another man's baby. Why should they, and why should I ruin my life?'

Because adoption is an option that can be considered at any time, both before and after the birth, it can be a fall-back position for a woman who wants to make a go of raising her child but who realizes that 'things are not going to work out'.

Tania, a 32-year-old teacher, was initially determined that she would raise her child as a single parent.

'I continued with the pregnancy because I wanted a child. For a long time I had a fantasy where I would find the right man, settle down, maybe get married, and have a family. But as the years go by you realize it isn't going to be quite like that. When I found out I was pregnant I was really pleased, even though it wasn't planned and I had split up with the father. I knew that this could be my one chance and if I waited for the big 'relationship' I might be too old to have a kid.

'My friends were sceptical but supportive, one even came to antenatal classes and was there at the birth, so I wasn't isolated and alone. But afterwards, when I was at home I felt really overwhelmed with what I had taken on. Peter didn't sleep well and cried all the time. I was really uptight (which made Peter worse). The health visitor talked a lot about post-natal depression, and maybe it was, but I just felt like I had made a really big mistake. I told myself things would get better but they didn't.

'A month after I came home with him I knew that, although I loved him, having that child was the most disastrous mistake I had made and I knew I was starting to resent him.

'I ended up phoning the Samaritans, not because I felt suicidal but because I had to talk to someone who didn't know me and wouldn't judge me. I sort of rehearsed how I felt with them and then talked to my health visitor who explained about fostering and adoption. For me it was the right thing, and I think it was for the baby too. I met the couple who were going to take him, and I'm glad about that. I gave them a letter for him when he's older, I can't imagine how I'd feel if I met him. I think about that a lot. I hope he'll understand.'

Opting for adoption

This is what happens if you decide to have your child adopted.

Before the birth

You don't have to tell anyone about your decision until after the birth, but it may make things easier if you discuss your intentions with your midwife. Your ante-natal care programme should be the same as if you are intending to keep your child, and you may find it quite an ordeal to meet with other women who are planning futures which will be so different. You are entitled to the same maternity benefits as every other pregnant woman, and if you are working you are entitled to the same maternity leave. You are not obliged to tell your employer that you intend to have your child adopted, although you may feel you wish to make this clear.

If you have been in contact with social services or an adoption agency, you will probably have already met 'your' social worker, and you may have discussed with them what kind of family you would like your child to grow up in. When the people who will adopt your child have been selected it may be possible for you to meet them. This can help you to imagine your child in his or her new home. If there is anything special that you would like the adoptive parents to know, the social worker can pass them on on your behalf. You may wish to write a letter and perhaps send a photograph of yourself.

Social services or the agency handling the adoption will want to interview you, and if possible, the man responsible for the pregnancy, to obtain the fullest possible information about you both and your families. This helps them to identify the most appropriate adoptive parents for your child, and also provides them with information which can be given to the adopters, for them to pass on to the child. If you are unmarried, and the father does not have parental responsibility for the child, his formal permission is not necessary for the adoption. However, the social worker is required by law to try to contact him if possible, both to hear what he thinks about the adoption and to collect information that your child may find useful later. *No one can force you to reveal the identity of the father unless you wish to do so.*

It is useful if the hospital at which the baby is born knows that you are planning to have the child adopted. Hospital practice varies; you may be given a choice about how much you want to see and care for your baby. Some hospitals may encourage you to look after the baby until you go home, but the final decision should be yours.

When you leave the hospital, usually about five days after the birth, the baby may be looked after by foster parents or may go straight to the adoptive parents. You will have discussed these arrangements with your social worker.

After the birth

You will be given every opportunity to change your mind about the adoption, and many women find that they have very mixed feelings, perhaps changing from day to day.

You cannot give formal agreement to the adoption until your baby is at least six weeks old. This is to allow you time to reflect on whether this is really what you want. If you change your mind during this time you would normally have the child returned to you, unless there are specific circumstances that would make the adoption agency worried about your ability to care for your child. The court cannot finalize the adoption until the baby has lived with its adopters for at least three months after that, and the adoption agency has provided the court with a report assuring it that all is well in the child's new home. Although it is still possible for you to change your mind about the adoption during this time, it is much more difficult to have the child returned to you, because the court would have to be convinced that such a move would be in the child's best interests.

There is a procedure called 'freeing for adoption' which you may wish to discuss with your social worker. This procedure enables your part of the adoption process (the formal giving of agreement) to be finalized even if for some reason your child has not yet settled in with a new family.

When the adoption order has been agreed by the court, the birth parents no longer have any legal relationship with, or responsibility for, the child.

The period after the birth can be a very difficult time. Friends and relatives may not know what to say or how to behave. Usually births are times of celebration where the mother is congratulated and because of this they may act quite inappropriately by ignoring everything that has happened and avoiding the subject.

After the adoption

Grief, loss, and anger are often felt by women after the adoption. These may be mixed with feelings of relief. Sometimes these emotions linger on long after the event. It often helps if you have someone with whom you can talk frankly about how you feel.

You may feel that you want to try to put the experience behind you, or you may wish to meet other women who have been through the same experiences, or you may wish to seek professional counselling. The organizations listed at the end of this book will be able to help.

If you wish to receive news about the progress of your child after the adoption, you should make this clear to your social workers so that the adopters can be asked to send information to the adoption agency or social services department (social work department in Scotland). Everyone needs to be clear about whether news will be passed on to you as soon as it is received or given to you if you ask. If letters cannot be safely sent to your home you may prefer to have them sent to someone you trust, such as a friend, solicitor, or social worker.

Your child's future

It is important to remember that the adoptive parents have the right to decide all issues concerning the child after adoption, such as where the family lives, and whether they have any further contact with the agency and people who arranged the adoption.

The adopters will have the responsibility of telling your child that she or he is adopted. But how and when they do this is entirely up to them.

After the adoption the child usually takes on the surname of the adoptive parents, and may even be given first names which are different from those you chose. The social worker does not have to tell you what these new names are.

You can write your child a letter to read when he or she is older to help them understand why they were adopted. This letter can be given to the adoptive parents and a copy can also be kept by the adoption agency or social work department. You can pass information about yourself to the agency at any time.

From the age of 18 (17 in Scotland) your daughter or son will have the right to ask for, and receive, a copy of their birth certificate. This shows the name you gave your child. Also she or he can usually find out which agency or social services department arranged the adoption. The statutory 'Adoption Contact Register' enables you to record a contact name and address which will be sent to your adult son or daughter if they decide to use the register to trace you.

These issues may seem very far away if you are only just now thinking about relinquishing a new baby for adoption, but it makes sense to consider them now even if you do not come to a decision.

Issues to consider

Emotional after-effects

Adoption is not an easy option. Studies have shown that giving up a baby is tremendously stressful for the birth mother, and it has been likened to having a 'still birth'. In fact one Australian study of 213 single mothers whose babies have been adopted[7] makes the case that it can be *even more* stressful than bereavement because the loss is 'self-inflicted' (a consequence of the mother's choice) and because the child continues to exist.

It is important to bear in mind that in this study, *half of the women responded well to the adoption and suffered no long-term adverse effects*, but many of those who adjusted less well compared the experience to the death of a child or a divorce. Half of these women experienced a persistent and increasing sense of loss over periods of up to 30 years, and they were more likely to suffer depression, anxiety, alcohol abuse, and physical ill health than single mothers who had kept their children. The sense of loss varied over time but tended to be particularly acute at key times, especially the child's birthday, the date the child started school, or reached eighteen. Family occasions and media coverage of topics related to adoption are also triggers of powerful feelings.

The key difference between the women who suffered badly from relinquishing their child and those who recovered well seemed to be the amount of support they received from those around them. Birth mothers who had supportive family and friends who would allow them to talk openly about the experience and made them feel loved and valued came through the experience much better.

Future contact

Years ago it was always assumed that there would be no contact between an adopted child and its birth mother. It was believed that it was best for all concerned that the break should be total and parents who placed a child for adoption usually did so on the understanding that the child would not have access to information other than their birth certificate.

Today it is thought that although adoption makes a child a full member of a new family, information about his or her origins may be important to them. There are some sound practical reasons for this. Every day we discover more about the consequences of our genetic inheritance. We now know that many serious illnesses, including some cancers, run in families. This means that unless an adopted person has access to the medical history of their birth parents they may miss out on information that could help them to safeguard their own health. Many children and adults who have been adopted are highly motivated to find out about their birth parents, who may be happy to be traced.

Adoptive parents are nowadays advised to tell children from an early age that they are adopted, and to give them as much information as possible about the birth parents without revealing their identity.

The Adoption Contact Register exists to put people and their birth parents or other relatives in touch with each other *when this is what they both want*. In Scotland a separate voluntary service called Birthlink deals with these enquiries, and the National Organisation for the Counselling of Adoptees and their Parents (NORCAP) also runs its own register (see p. 144).

A relative who wishes to be included on the register has to prove that they are related to the adopted person. Sometimes birth mothers may wish to use a contact address other than their own, usually that of a friend or relative, or an organization or individual such as a counsellor or social worker.

The way that attitudes have changed towards contact between adopted children and their birth parents over recent years has transformed the meaning of adoption because even if the individuals involved choose not to make contact they are aware that the possibility of contact exists. This can sometimes help to ease pain but, in certain circumstances, it can increase it. Before the registers were established a birth mother who longed to meet her child could always fantasize that their child was searching for them too. A birth mother who leaves information about herself with a register and is not contacted may feel rejected, as may someone who has been adopted and who finds his or her birth mother has decided not to register her details.

Sharing the knowledge

It can be extremely difficult for a birth mother to decide whether to share the knowledge about the existence of her adopted child with friends, family, and future partners.

For past generations there was an unwritten rule that such things were simply not discussed. Adoption was stigmatized, but it was stigmatized in the context that the sex which had resulted in the pregnancy was immoral and sinful. In effect, sex was stigmatized more than the adoption. If a woman was pregnant, what else could she do? Today, curiously, sex outside marriage is accepted but adoption is still stigmatized, although the stigma is accorded for different reasons.

Some people, often those whose lives are untouched by the problems of accidental pregnancies, see women who proceed with pregnancies and then relinquish the child for adoption as 'callous' or 'hard'. It is commonly observed that giving up a baby after the experience of pregnancy and childbirth is more 'unnatural' than terminating the pregnancy, especially in its earliest stages.

These judgements are often made by people looking at adoption as an abstract issue rather than in the context of a very specific situation. Those who make sweeping negative comments about adoption similarly fail to place themselves in the situation of the women for whom the decision is the least undesirable of a number of undesirable options. In any case, many other people regard mothers who give up their babies as 'heroic', 'compassionate', and 'selfless'.

Whether she wishes to or not, a woman's circumstances may force her to offer some explanation to family, friends, and colleagues about the outcome of the pregnancy. It is not easy to conceal a pregnancy in its final months and, while some women find it easier to evade the issue, perhaps even by claiming that the child was stillborn—a situation which the birth mother may feel more comfortable in disclosing because it tends to elicit unconditional sympathy rather than the confused reaction that many people have when confronted with adoption. Most women find it easier to explain their decision on a 'need to know' basis.

Women who conceal that they have relinquished a child for adoption are often extremely concerned that a future partner, or subsequent children, will discover their secret. There are, of course, no guarantees that this will not happen. Even if a woman avoids any contact with the agencies involved and forwards no details to the contact register, a highly motivated individual prepared to engage in a considerable amount of detective work may be able to trace her. There are no absolute safeguards to protect against this. But a woman can be confident that should she decide to keep her situation a secret, she will not be betrayed by doctors, social workers, or any of the agencies with whom she has contact.

It is unlikely that the proportion of women with unplanned pregnancies who chose adoption will increase significantly. But the very fact that adoptive parents are encouraged to discuss the birth parents with their adopted child give the birth mother a place in the child's life. For many women this greater openness will make what is often seen as the most difficult choice a realistic option.

References

1. Sally MacIntyre (1977). *Single and pregnant.* Croom Helm, London.
2. Michael Schofield (1965). *The sexual behaviour of young people.* Longman, London.
3. Bouchier, P., Lambert, L., and Tiseliotis, J. (1991). *Parting with a child for adoption,* p. 29. British Agencies for Adoption and Fostering, London.
4. Howe, D., Sabridge, P., and Hinings, D. (1992). *Half a million women: mothers who lose their children by adoption.* Penguin, London.
5. Jean Pochin (1969). *Without a wedding ring: casework with unmarried parents.* Constable, London.
6. Joss Shawyer (1979). *Death by adoption.* Cicada Press, New Zealand. *And* Sorosky, A.D., Baran, A., and Pannor, R. (1978). *The adoption triangle.* Anchor Press/Doubleday, New York, NY.
7. Winkler, R. and van Keppel, M. (1984). *Relinquishing mothers in adoption: their long term adjustment.* Institute of Family Studies, Melbourne, Australia.

6

Considering motherhood

An unplanned pregnancy is not necessarily an unwanted pregnancy, and even those that are initially undesired may become wanted as they progress. It is not possible to generalize about why some women decide to keep their children and others do not. Women's decisions about pregnancy reflect the broader circumstances of their lives. The fact that, according to a recent report on unplanned pregnancy[1], marriage is an important factor in determining whether a woman with an unplanned pregnancy continues it or has an abortion, may reflect the fact that for many couples marriage implies a permanent commitment and consequently a suitable environment into which to bring a child. Often couples marry with the intention of 'starting a family soon'. An accidental pregnancy in this situation may simply mean bringing such a decision forward.

Society generally views motherhood as the natural, even inevitable, consequence of a stable partnership. A pregnancy within marriage is generally greeted with congratulations; outside marriage it is greeted with concern and sometimes even condemnation. A married woman who is ambivalent about the pregnancy may feel swept along by the way that people around her respond to her situation, or even how she thinks they will respond.

Stephanie, a 24-year-old bank clerk found that her parents greeted her unplanned pregnancy with relief.

> 'It wasn't just that they were delighted, they were relieved. We had been married for four years and I think they thought there was a problem, although we had just decided that we wanted to spend some time together on our own before starting a family. In some ways it was as though mum didn't regard us as being properly married until I told her I was pregnant.'

Amanda, pregnant as a result of what she describes as a 'casual liaison' with a colleague faced very mixed reactions:

'When I found I was pregnant I went into shock. You have to understand I had no relationship with the father, nor did I want one. We had had sex because we were travelling together, we fancied each other, and to be honest it was more convenient to sleep together than not. But that was the end of it. Yet I did want the baby.

'Everybody said I was insane, but I thought about it long and hard and I was sure I could handle it. I'm self reliant, I make enough money to support myself and a child. My job is sufficiently flexible to allow me to work at home a lot. And, if I'm honest, I'm just plain broody. I'm 36 now and the way I look at it I can either wait on the chance that I *may* meet the right guy to get pregnant by or I can go for it now.

'The only person who approves of what I'm doing is my best friend and maybe it's significant that she and her partner can't have children. Her attitude is that if you look at all the young girls who manage to have kids with no education, no home, and no income, mine should have it made—father or no father.

'My doctor was an utter bastard. He assumed I would want an abortion and gave me a lecture on responsibility and the problems faced by children who are emotionally neglected by their parents. My own mum and dad were nearly as bad. I think my mother's first comment was that she hoped I wasn't assuming that they would look after the child while I went skiing.'

Pat found that the reactions of her friends and colleagues were particularly shaped by the fact that her partner was younger than she was.

'Steve was just 23, I was 27 but I had already had one ectopic pregnancy and I felt that if I didn't have this child I might not have another chance. Anyway, I was confident that Steve would be OK and that even if he left me I could manage.

'My friends seemed to see it as a matter of when Steve would leave me rather than if. One even said to me that I should start planning from the beginning as if I was going to be a single mother. Everyone's attitude was that men are more immature than women and that he'd resent having to play the father while his mates were off at the football. That was four years ago. We're still together, happy, and Mark now has a sister. Of course there have been tensions. But if truth be known, I have been the one who has found it most difficult to balance being a parent with all the other things in my life—Steve just seems to have rolled with it.'

Today, unmarried women have more freedom to choose to both have children and remain socially accepted than at any time in British history. Women who become pregnant outside traditional family arrangements are no longer vilified, banished to the workhouse and seen as morally corrupt. Single parents run one in five British households[2], and although most of these will be single as a consequence of divorce or widowhood, many women have always taken sole responsibility for their children.

While traditional Conservatives panic about the decline of the traditional family, most of society seems to accept that family structures have changed and that the single-parent family can be a legitimate alternative to the traditional two-parent family unit. Even those who are horrified by the concept of single parents in general, are forced to concede that many single parents raise their children in an exemplary manner.

The prevalence of single parenthood amongst the 'respectable middle classes' has meant that when conservative politicians raise concerns about what they perceive to be the breakdown of the family, they tend to isolate particular groups of single parents as problematic: usually those who are dependent on state welfare. 'Dependence' is seen by many as the greater problem.

Curiously, in recent years, it is women who have become *deliberately pregnant*, rather than accidentally pregnant, outside traditional family arrangements who have attracted the greatest amount of moral condemnation. Conservative politicians have railed against young, single women who become pregnant deliberately to obtain welfare payments and priority housing. Women who choose to become pregnant, despite the fact that they have no partner, perhaps taking advantage of assisted conception techniques to do so, are also seen as a cause of official consternation. The focus of concern seems to have subtly altered to target those who consciously reject traditional family arrangements rather than those who accidentally find themselves outside of them.[3]

How much family planning do you really *need*?

Much of the concern about *accidental* pregnancy comes from health promotion agencies concerned with reproductive health issues, such as the Family Planning Association and the Health Education Authority, who place great emphasis on the need to 'plan pregnancy' to maximize the chances of a healthy outcome for both mother and child.

Preparation for a new baby is obviously important, and by planning the timing of a pregnancy a woman can maximize her control over her situation both during the pregnancy and afterwards. An ideal situation might be for a woman to look at her diary over the coming 18 months and decide on the most convenient month for her to give birth. She might wish to weigh up 'serious' issues (such as whether she can arrange child care for existing children) or 'trivial' issues (such as an even spread of birthdays throughout the year). Several months before her intended conception she might embark on a serious programme of preparation for pregnancy: healthy eating, exercise to tone her body, appropriate vitamin supplements. She might already set money aside to ease possible financial difficulties and even start planning her work so as to allow it to be easily delegated to others when she takes maternity leave.

Planning in any area of life gives the planner an advantage. The motto 'be prepared' is not only relevant to boy scouts!

By planning your pregnancy, you have the chance to prepare

- your own health
- practical arrangements
- your relationship so that it is able to cope with the strains of parenthood
- your own state of mind.

However, there is a huge difference between what is ideal, or even desirable, and what is *strictly necessary*. In ordinary circumstances, there is no reason for a woman to worry that she will be inadequately prepared if her pregnancy is unplanned—nine months is quite long enough to make plans and adjust to the situation. Nor should she fear that she has put the pregnancy at risk—only in the rarest cases would this be so.

For the most part, an unplanned pregnancy is little different to a planned one, and there are dozens of books offering comprehensive advice and information on pregnancy. This chapter looks at some of the issues of particular concern to women who unexpectedly find themselves facing the knowledge that they are on the road to motherhood.

Preconception and antenatal care

The concept of antenatal care has been a part of medicine from the turn of the century. As early as 1901, the Scottish obstetrician, J. W. Ballantyne proposed a 'pre-maternity hospital' where women could be cared for and doctors could study the pregnant state. Over the next three decades antenatal care became increasingly widespread with 80 per cent of women receiving some kind of antenatal care by 1935.[4] However, at that time and until recent decades, antenatal care concentrated on maintaining the health of the woman, rather than considering the developing fetus. Little was known about what could or could not influence fetal development. In fact it was not until the thalidomide tragedy in the late 1950s and early 1960s when hundreds of women gave birth to severely disabled babies after taking the anti-emetic drug Distaval that the medical profession recognized that substances taken in pregnancy could cross the placenta and harm the fetus.

Since then much attention has been given to what can and cannot harm a developing pregnancy. Medical science has also revealed that the health of a baby is not only affected by the actions of his mother while pregnant, but even by what she does before he is conceived. *Preconception care* is now a recognized part of reproductive health care and this can be a great cause of anxiety to women who find that they are pregnant without having followed the appropriate advice.

Marianne became pregnant at 34 quite naturally, after trying to conceive for more than seven years. She and her partner had gone through four cycles of failed IVF and they had reconciled themselves to childlessness.

'Once I got over the shock, I started to freak out a bit. This pregnancy was so precious yet I had done everything wrong. When we finished the IVF treatment we deliberately decided that we would stop living as though I was about to get pregnant. I stopped taking folic acid supplements and I was drinking far more alcohol than I should. The months before I tested positive I had even been on a low-calorie, low-fat diet because I had decided that if I wasn't going to be pregnant at least I was going to make the most of my body. What's more (you won't believe this) I had even had some dental X-rays taken. When the dentist asked me if I might be pregnant I had just laughed. Fortunately my doctor was very reassuring and calmed me down a lot.'

The fear that she may have unwittingly done something to damage her child is extremely common among women with unplanned pregnancies. While not wishing to trivialize the importance of pre-conception care, it is important to get the risks into perspective.

Preconception care

There are sound reasons why preconception care is important. A summary of evidence considered by the Parliamentary Health Committee in 1991[5] identified the following factors known to influence the outcome of a pregnancy: smoking, alcohol intake, medicines and recreational drugs, diet, infections such as rubella, toxoplasmosis and sexually transmitted infections, and exposure to environmental factors such as radiation and chemicals.

Today, women trying to conceive are advised to modify their behaviour at least three months prior to conception to achieve prime conditions for the start of pregnancy.

In particular women are advised to follow these guidelines.

- Cut down on drinks which contain caffeine, such as coffee, tea, and colas, as there is a slight risk that caffeine may affect fetal development. There is also some evidence to suggest that a high caffeine intake in the months prior to pregnancy may increase the risk of miscarriage.

- Ensure a balanced diet, and discuss whether or not you require vitamin supplements with your doctor. Vitamins are an issue of particular concern. Women are now advised to take 0.4 milligrams (400 micrograms) of folic acid a day for three months before conception until the twelfth week of pregnancy to reduce the risk of neural tube defects such as spina bifida. Women planning a pregnancy are also advised to avoid Vitamin A supplements as a high intake of Vitamin A has been linked to fetal defects.

- Give up smoking, as smokers tend to have lower birth-weight babies and smoking can cause problems with the way that the placenta functions.

- Cut down on alcohol intake, as alcohol is thought to increase the risk of miscarriage and the intake of large quantities of alcohol has been linked to the risk of fetal malformation.

- Have a blood test to check immunity to rubella (German Measles). If a woman is not immune most doctors will recommend inoculation against it as the disease can cause fetal damage. Likewise, some doctors test for toxoplasmosis.

- Have a smear test, and possibly a check for chlamydia or other vaginal infections. A breast check may also be suggested.

Obviously, once a woman knows she is pregnant, if she intends to have the baby, it makes sense for her to follow advice which will maximize her chance of having a healthy baby.

Usually there is absolutely no cause for worry. For thousands of years, women have given birth to healthy babies without taking special precautions either before they conceived, or even when they knew they were pregnant. Embryos and fetuses are remarkably well protected as women who have tried to end their own pregnancies have often found out to their cost. Before the legalization of abortion women frequently damaged their own health with instruments or by taking substances thought to have abortion-inducing properties only to be delivered, eventually, of a perfectly healthy baby.

The resilience of pregnancies is also illustrated by the fact that things which are considered hazardous to pregnancy in our culture are considered to be perfectly acceptable, even recommended, in others. In her fascinating account of birth traditions[6], sociologist Jacqueline Vincent Priya, describes how different societies recommend different diets to pregnant women. For instance, pregnant Yoruba women in Africa are not encouraged to eat protein foods such as meat or fish, which is the opposite of advice given to pregnant women in developed societies. In many places, such as Bangladesh, pregnant women are encouraged not to eat too much so that their baby will be small and born without difficulties. Clearly, a large 'bonny' baby which we would regard as healthy can be a disaster in a society where women do not have access to a sophisticated obstetric service.

Often women's doubts and fears concentrate on the issues of contraception, drug use, and diet.

About contraception

There is no evidence to suggest that if a woman becomes pregnant whilst she is using a hormonal contraceptive (the pill, implants, or injections) the future baby will be affected. Thousands of babies have been conceived while their mothers were using the pill to no ill effect whatsoever, and the effect of pill usage on the developing pregnancy has been studied carefully.

In 1991, a study of more than 56 000 early pregnancies identified that 350 women had continued to take the pill while pregnant and concluded that 'oral contraceptive use is not associated with the development of major malformations'. It did identify a small increase in the risk of an abnormality of the arch of the foot, but as only two cases of this were found the authors of the study resolved that further studies would be needed to clarify whether this was, in fact, significant.[7]

If a woman with an IUD becomes pregnant and wishes to remain so, her doctor will recommend the removal of the device if he or she can still see the threads of the IUD passing through the cervix. If the threads are not visible the device would usually be left in place. Pregnancies with an IUD *in situ* are more prone miscarry.

Emergency contraception has been a subject of much debate. Some doctors insist that if a woman takes emergency contraceptive pills she should have an abortion if they fail and she becomes pregnant because the risk of abnormality is high. Setting aside the fact that no doctor can insist that a woman has an abortion for any reason, there is no evidence to show that babies born after their mother has used emergency contraception have a higher than usual incidence of abnormality. Doctors are cautious because the number of women who have continued pregnancies after using emergency contraception is quite small (the pregnancy clearly wasn't wanted, the woman was highly motivated to prevent it, and most women in this unfortunate situation have the pregnancy terminated), and they do not want to jump to a hasty conclusion. The Royal College of Obstetricians and Gynaecologists is currently maintaining a register of such cases.

About drugs

Some drugs taken in pregnancy cross the placenta and enter the fetal blood stream. This means that, if a woman takes certain drugs at particular stages of pregnancy, there is a risk of abnormalities or retarded growth. Many drugs are known to have adverse effects in pregnancy, many others are known to be safe, but in a large number of cases there is no firm evidence to decide on risk or safety. Quite understandably, the routine trials that are carried out to determine the safety of medicines for the general population usually exclude pregnant women. As a consequence, most pharmaceutical companies tend to 'play safe' and unless there is convincing evidence to suggest that the drug is definitely safe they will include a warning against use in pregnancy.

Any woman who knows she is pregnant, or is trying to conceive, should consult a doctor or pharmacist before taking any medicine. They should be able to assess the potential risks and benefits as they affect an individual woman.

Often the element of risk is more complicated than it seems. If, for example, a woman is suffering severely from a condition such as hay fever, is unable to sleep, and is severely stressed, a doctor may decide her condition is more likely to adversely affect the pregnancy than if she takes a particularly effective antihistamine.

If you are unexpectedly pregnant, and you discover that you have been taking a drug which carries a warning, or contraindication, against taking it in pregnancy, don't panic, but do tell your doctor so that he or she can assess any risk and reassure or advise you. Even if a drug is known to cause adverse affects at *some* stage in pregnancy, it may not be a problem at your current stage of pregnancy.

Depending on the stage of pregnancy in which they are taken, drugs can have different effects on the woman or the fetus or both. The first three months are the most critical, as drugs taken at this time may affect the development of the fetal organs leading to a congenital malformation. From the fourth to the sixth month some drugs may retard the growth of the fetus and cause the baby to have a low birth-weight. During the last three months some drugs can cause breathing difficulties in the new-born baby and can affect labour, causing it to be premature, delayed, or prolonged.

About diet

Health officials suggest that a woman should pay particular attention to a diet during pregnancy to avoid infections which could harm the pregnancy.

In particular women are advised to avoid certain ripened cheeses such as camembert, brie and blue-veined cheeses, paté, and ready-to-eat meats especially pre-cooked chicken (unless served piping hot) as these may contain bacteria which can lead to listeriosis—a flu-like illness which can lead to miscarriage, stillbirth, or severe illness in the new-born baby.

Poultry and raw meat and eggs (unless cooked until solid) can harbour salmonella, a form of food poisoning. And goat's milk, unwashed vegetables, and salads can carry toxoplasmosis, which may be symptomless in the woman but cause a range of problems for the fetus. Toxoplasmosis is most commonly passed on through cats' faeces, so pregnant or about-to-be pregnant women are advised to avoid contact with litter trays.

It is important to note that these diseases are *extremely rare*, and the chance of contracting one from an occasional chicken salad is remote.

Pregnant women are also advised to cut liver products, such as paté, out of their diet because liver is a rich source of vitamin A which in large quantities is associated with birth defects. And for three months before and after conception they are advised to take supplements of 0.4 mg folic acid, one of the B vitamins which offers some protection against neural tube defects such as spina bifida.

When you discover you have an unplanned pregnancy, your best course of action is to start following the appropriate dietary advice from the day you realize you are pregnant. There is no point in raking over the past to identify moments which might have increased the risk to the pregnancy. The overwhelming likelihood is that all is well.

Too old or too young?

Women often worry about whether they are too old or too young to have a child There is of course no categorical answer to this because so much rests on a woman's attitude to pregnancy and motherhood. Some young women at 17 are more able and responsible than others at 30. If a woman is capable of conceiving and carrying a pregnancy to term, she is probably capable of bringing a healthy child into the world. The biggest risks faced by older women are reduced fertility (obviously not a problem in the case of an unplanned pregnancy), increased risk of miscarriage, and fetal abnormality. Some studies have also shown that older women are at greater risk of ectopic pregnancy and some pregnancy related conditions such as diabetes and high blood-pressure[8]. However, the risk of such problems can often be circumvented by medical attention.

Within the fertile age-range, the age at which it is considered best to have a child changes with fashion. During the last decade, the number of children born in England and Wales each year to women in their early 20s fell by 15 000, while the number born to women in their early 30s rose by 30 000.[9]

Despite this, doctors still refer to any woman having her first baby over the age of 35 as an 'elderly primagravida' which can make some women feel as if they must be doing something abnormal and perhaps placing themselves and their future child at risk. Usually this is not the case. How successfully a woman adapts to a surprise motherhood has more to do with her temperament, her relationship, and her life-style than her biological age.

If a woman is planning a pregnancy she is in a position to weigh up carefully whether the time is right for her to have a child. A woman with an unplanned pregnancy has to weigh up the pros and cons of her situation quite quickly. Each woman's situation is different. There is no 'right time' to have a child. There are advantages and disadvantages at every age.

The pros and cons of having a child

In your early 20s

Pros
- you'll still be young as your child grows up
- you'll probably suffer less from tiredness during pregnancy
- you're less likely to have complications like high blood-pressure
- you'll probably recover from childbirth quickly and regain your figure faster
- the child's grandparents are likely to be still young.

Cons
- you may resent giving up your freedom to socialize
- you may not yet have established a career pattern
- you will have had less time to save to see you through lean times ahead
- you may feel more intimidated by older doctors and midwives
- if your partner is the same age, he may find it difficult to adjust to the responsibilities of fatherhood.

In your late 20s

Pros
- you are probably more confident and knowledgeable about your body than when you were younger, so you may be more at ease when you are pregnant
- you may be more financially secure
- you may be more confident about your partner
- you may be more confident about what *you* want and need

Cons
- it may be difficult to take a career break as you may have long-term financial commitments, such as a mortgage
- you may feel that you are being pushed into motherhood because people expect it of you at this age
- you may feel that motherhood isolates you from your childless friends.

In your early 30s

Pros

- you probably feel more confident and assertive than you did in your 20s
- you have had more time to be sure that you want a child
- you may be more financially stable
- you are more likely to have other mothers among your friends who can give you support

Cons

- your labour might be a little longer than it would have been in your 20s
- it may be more of a struggle to stay fit during your pregnancy
- it may take you slightly longer to recover from the birth and to regain your figure

In your late 30s

Pros

- you will be more experienced in life and more mature
- if your partner is the same age he may also be more able to cope with the stress of living with a pregnant woman
- you will have had the chance to 'let your hair down' before the responsibility of motherhood
- you are probably more financially secure than when you were younger
- you may have been able to establish yourself in your career and consequently have more control over the way you work.

Cons

- you have an increased risk of bearing a child with a disability (see pp. 128–49)
- you are more likely to be at risk of high blood-pressure and varicose veins during pregnancy
- you may feel out of place at the antenatal clinic if all the other women are younger
- you and your partner may have become set in your ways and so find it difficult to adjust to the baby

- your parents may be very elderly and find it difficult to enjoy their grandchild
- your friends may find it hard to share your concerns if their children are significantly older

In your 40s

Pros

- you may find it easier to be assertive and to find out information from medical staff
- you may be more financially settled
- if you have children already, they may now be old enough to look after themselves or even to help you with the baby
- at the antenatal classes, mixing with women who are half your age will put you in touch with a younger generation

Cons

- you may have a more difficult birth
- you are more likely to suffer from complications in pregnancy, such as high blood-pressure
- your labour is likely to be longer and more exhausting
- you have a significantly higher risk of bearing a child with a disability
- your child is likely to lose his or her grandparents at an early age.

Worries about disability

Older women often fear that, although they would dearly love to have the child from an accidental pregnancy, the risk of abnormality is too high for them to take the chance.

It is important to get these risks into perspective.

Almost every woman runs the risk of having a child with a disability, regardless of her age or whether there is any previous history of genetic disease in the family, because almost everyone carries one or more recessively inherited genetic defects. Many abnormal pregnancies are conceived, although most miscarry, often very early in the pregnancy. Although maternal age is a significant factor as can be seen from the following table[10] (and there is some controversy about whether or not paternal age plays a part), the majority of children with genetic disabilities are born to fit, healthy parents. This is even true of Down's syndrome which is often associated with 'older mothers'. The majority of Down's syndrome babies are born to mothers under 35, but statistically the risk to younger women is less because more of them are having children.

Age of woman	Risk of Down's syndrome	Risk of other chromosome defect
20	1 in 1923	1 in 526
25	1 in 1205	1 in 476
30	1 in 885	1 in 384
35	1 in 365	1 in 178
40	1 in 109	1 in 63
45	1 in 32	1 in 18

Whether the pregnancy is planned or unplanned, women who fear that their child may be at risk of genetic abnormality are usually offered a range of tests. As most of these cannot be carried out until the later stages of the pregnancy, a woman who only realizes that she is pregnant in the third or fourth month is often in exactly the same position as a woman who identified her pregnancy in its earliest stages.

It's up to you

No woman should be forced to have any test which she does not want to have and it is up to you to decide what, if any, action you take on the basis of the results. You may wish to discuss the options with your doctor or midwife, or with your partner, family, or friends, before the tests are taken.

If the test shows that your baby would be born with a serious disability, you should be offered the choice of whether or not to continue with the pregnancy. It may be better for you to consider what you would want to do before the test, but you do not have to make up your mind in advance. Even if you are sure that you would not wish to consider an abortion, you may still want to have the tests. It can either reassure you that your child is likely to be born healthy, or it will give you time to prepare for having a baby with special needs.

The following methods can be used to detect fetal handicap.

Amniocentesis

Amniocentesis is routinely offered to pregnant women over the age of 35. It can be used to detect many chromosomal abnormalities including Tay-Sachs disease and Down's syndrome. The procedure involves taking fluid from the sac which surrounds the baby through a needle inserted through the abdominal wall and guided by ultrasound. Cells from the fetus, which are present in the amniotic fluid are then tested for chromosomal abnormalities.

Amniocentesis cannot be carried out until the fifteenth or sixteenth week of the pregnancy as before then the amniotic sac is too small for the fluid to be extracted safely. It usually takes two to three weeks for the results to be processed.

Amniocentesis is an extremely safe procedure, but there is a slight risk (about one in 100) of triggering a miscarriage. The miscarriage risk is why amniocentesis tests are usually only routinely offered to women over the age of 35. If the woman is under 35, and neither partner has a family history of genetic problems' the risk of miscarriage is probably greater than the risk of uncovering a genetic abnormality. For older women, the risk of discovering an abnormality is greater than the risk of miscarriage.

Chorion Villus Sampling (CVS)

CVS involves the analysis of a small piece of tissue from the placenta. Because the fetus and the placenta both develop from the same initial cells, a genetic abnormality in the fetal cells is likely to be present in the placenta. The cells are gathered through a small tube which is passed through the cervix, or by inserting a needle (guided by ultrasound) through the abdominal wall. The cells are then tested for abnormalities.

CVS can be carried out earlier than amniocentesis, usually between the ninth and eleventh week, but it carries a slightly higher risk of triggering a miscarriage.

Maternal blood tests

In later pregnancy it is possible to detect some of the proteins produced by the fetus in the woman's blood. If a pregnant woman has raised levels of a chemical called alphafoetolprotein (AFP) in her blood it may indicate that the fetus is likely to have a spinal cord defect such as spina bifida, a lower than usual level may indicate other abnormalities. If this test shows abnormal levels the woman would probably be advised to have an amniocentesis to confirm the diagnosis. This test can be carried out between 15 and 18 weeks' gestation. Some hospitals routinely carry out AFP tests, others do not but should be able to provide it on request.

Tripe test ('Barts test')

Women carrying a fetus with Down's syndrome are more likely to have a higher than normal level of the pregnancy hormone hCG, a lower than normal level of AFP and a higher than normal level of a hormone called oestriol. These factors, considered with her age, will indicate whether the pregnancy falls into a high-risk category.

Through a simple blood test, specialists can determine whether a woman matches this profile and is therefore likely to have an affected pregnancy. These women can then be offered amniocentesis to confirm the diagnosis. The triple test is sometimes offered to women who would not routinely be offered an amniocentesis test, perhaps because they are in their 20s.

The test is usually carried out when the pregnancy is at 16 to 18 weeks' gestation, and the results take just a few days.

Ultrasound

Ultrasound examinations can reveal certain defects of the spinal cord and abnormalities of the head and the heart. However, these are very difficult to spot until the pregnancy is quite advanced—usually at about 18 to 19 weeks.

Chordocentesis (fetal blood sampling)

A needle guided by ultrasound is used to take a small sample of blood from the umbilical cord. The cells are then tested as they are in CVS, but because fetal blood cells are taken the results can be obtained more quickly. This risk of miscarriage is similar to that in CVS.

Fetoscopy

Certain rare liver and skin diseases can be detected by examining the fetus with a special telescope-like instrument which is inserted into the uterus.

Coping with pregnancy

Once a woman with an unplanned pregnancy has decided to have her baby, whether it was planned or unplanned becomes irrelevant. The arrangements for antenatal care, for maternity allowances and benefits' and for maternity leave from work are exactly the same— whether the pregnancy is accidental or the result of years of trying, whether the woman lives with a partner or is single.

Every bookshop and library has shelves of books providing advice for pregnant mothers (and fathers). Here we will only cover the aspects of maternity care about which you may be particularly worried if your pregnancy is a surprise.

Arranging antenatal care

Throughout the pregnancy, every woman is entitled to receive antenatal care either at a hospital or antenatal clinic, or with her own GP or a community midwife. It is important that women with unplanned pregnancies, 'get into the system' quite quickly, so as to take advantage of the health care offered.

Most women have their first, and longest, antenatal check up between the eighth and twelfth week of pregnancy, and it is generally accepted that the earlier a woman attends the better it is.

At the initial antenatal appointment, the doctor will usually seek answers to questions about the following.

- The state of the woman's general health, including past operations or illnesses, pregnancies, or miscarriages.
- Information about inherited illness in either the woman's family or that of her partner. This is to determine any specific risk of genetic illnesses.

- Ethnic origin. This is because some inherited illness are more common among specific ethnic groups.
- The woman's menstrual cycle, including details of last period, to allow the doctor to estimate the date of delivery.

The woman is weighed, and her weight gain will usually be checked regularly. Most women will put on between 10 to 12.5 kilos (22 to 28 lbs) in pregnancy—most of it after week 20.

A woman's height is usually measured on the first visit because height gives a rough guide to the size of a woman's pelvis. Some small women have especially small pelvises and may need to consider whether a caesarean section delivery is an appropriate option.

A blood test will be taken to check blood group and rhesus status, whether she is anaemic, immune to rubella, has a disease such as syphilis or hepatitis B which may cause problems if not treated. Women are not routinely tested for HIV during pregnancy.

If your unplanned pregnancy happened as a result of unprotected sex with someone other than a regular partner and you think you may have risked HIV infection, you may wish to ask your doctor for the opportunity to discuss HIV testing and counselling.

A doctor may carry out an internal examination, to feel the size of the uterus, and thus confirm the gestational age of the pregnancy. This will be particularly important if you are not certain when you conceived. Often women are surprised to discover that the pregnancy is further advanced than they believed.

After the first antenatal visit, most women will be asked to attend appointments every month until the last two or three months of pregnancy when the appointments become more frequent.

At each antenatal visit the woman's urine will be checked for sugar and proteins which may indicate problems which require treatment. Some women develop diabetes in pregnancy ('gestational diabetes'). Her blood pressure will also be examined as, in later pregnancy, high blood pressure can be dangerous to the woman and the pregnancy.

Pregnant women are usually encouraged to attend antenatal classes in the last eight to ten weeks before the baby is due. These cover issues such as:

- health in pregnancy
- what happens during labour and birth
- coping with labour and information about pain relief
- exercises to keep fit during pregnancy and to help you in labour
- relaxation
- caring for the new-born baby, including feeding
- the woman's health after birth.

Antenatal classes provide pregnant women with an opportunity to meet each other, get to know some of the professionals involved in their care and to discuss any worries. Many welcome partners or friends. Some health authorities run classes specially for younger women who may feel out of place at the standard classes.

It is important to remember that although it is sensible for a woman to take full advantage of all the antenatal services on offer, women have been having babies for hundreds of years with no antenatal care or checks whatsoever, and this is still the case in many parts of the world. A woman who discovers her pregnancy, or who decides to keep her pregnancy, at a comparatively late gestational age, may have missed out on some helpful advice and she may have less time in which to find out how the maternity care system works, to get to know the professionals involved, to consider whether or not she wants tests, or to decide on her favoured delivery arrangements—but she is unlikely to have done anything to put her pregnancy at risk.

Being pregnant

Pregnancy inevitably causes major changes in a woman's life. If the pregnancy is planned, there will have been time to mull these over in advance. However when the pregnancy is accidental some of the changes may catch a woman by surprise.

Changes to your health

The changes to a woman's health are the same whether the pregnancy was planned or unplanned. Some women seem to sail through pregnancy remaining active until they go into labour. For others it is nine months of agony. Most women experience something in between. The only thing that is certain is that you will not be able to predict how you will feel, nor what you will be capable of doing during the pregnancy.

A trouble-free first pregnancy does not guarantee an easy second pregnancy, and conversely if a woman suffers severe morning-sickness during a first pregnancy it does not mean she will have the same problem second time around.

If you are worried by any symptoms of pregnancy, at any time, it is best to discuss the problem with your doctor or midwife.

Changes at work

Every woman has to make her own decision about how much to tell her employer and colleagues about her pregnancy. There are some advantages in announcing the pregnancy.

- If you are struggling because of tiredness and morning sickness, your employers may be more sympathetic if they know there is 'a good reason', and that you have not suddenly become sloppy and disinterested in your work.
- Your employers may be grateful to know your situation early so that they have plenty of time to make adequate arrangements for your maternity leave cover.
- You will be able to discuss your future plans with your colleagues.

On the other hand, you may have concerns in disclosing the information.

- You may be worried that they will disapprove of your situation and try to put pressure on you to end the pregnancy.
- If your employers are particularly underhand, they may try to take steps to avoid paying you maternity benefit.

Rights at work

Your rights at work depend on the size of the company you work for, and the length of time you have been employed by them. Broadly, you should have the right to return to work and/or to receive statutory maternity pay from your employer, but there are certain circumstances in which these rights do not apply. The Citizen's Advice Bureau and trade unions (if there is one at the workplace) or your personnel officer are good sources of advice.

Changes to your finances

Having a child has serious financial consequences. However generous a woman's maternity arrangements at work, it inevitably means her income is reduced at just the time she has increased expenditure to prepare for the new baby.

State benefits are rather paltry, but they can alleviate some of the hardship and it makes sense to take advantage of them. Leaflets outlining the available benefits are usually available in post offices, libraries, and GP surgeries.

All women have the right to free dental treatment on the NHS while pregnant and for a year after birth. Prescriptions for NHS medicines are also free during pregnancy, and for the year following the birth. Once the pregnancy has been confirmed, the doctor or midwife issues a form which is sent to the local Family Health Service Authority who, in turn, send an exemption certificate back to the pregnant women.

Pregnant women on income support can also claim:

- free milk tokens
- free vitamin tablets during pregnancy and while breast feeding, and free vitamin drops for the child until he or she is five.
- vouchers for glasses
- fares to and from hospital
- a lump sum maternity payment.

All mothers are entitled to claim child benefit, regardless of their income.

Changes in your relationships

Even when a pregnancy is planned and wanted it can be a deeply unsettling time for both partners. During pregnancy and after the birth it is common for each partner to find it hard to cope with conflicting demands and responsibilities. Men often feel pushed to one side and neglected as attention is focused on the pregnancy and then the baby, while women frequently find it difficult to respond as a lover and friend when their days are so dominated by motherhood.

The tensions may be exacerbated if the pregnancy is unplanned and the male partner has some reservations about fatherhood.

Julia, a 27-year-old hairdresser, found that her partner seemed to retreat from the relationship at first:

'I thought he'd be quite happy about it. We'd been living together for three years and when we'd talked about having a baby he had seemed keen. But when I told him that I thought I was pregnant he assumed that I'd have an abortion. When I explained that I wanted his child he really freaked out. It was as though he had never thought about what it meant and suddenly the enormity hit him.

'We eventually worked it through but for a week I thought I was going to have to choose between him and the baby. Mind you, when he came round he got into it in a really big way. By the time Jenni was born he knew more about obstetrics than the midwives!'

Sue, a 25-year-old teacher found her partner's reaction was very different to that which she had expected.

'Peter's first words were: "Oh no!" even though he insisted he was happy about it. Then it was as though he was trying to pretend it wasn't happening. Every time I tried to talk about the baby he would change the subject. I couldn't get him to plan at all. Then when I got to three months he changed and really started to get into it. I think he was really scared at first and he needed to get used to the idea.'

Some men can find the idea of pregnancy quite terrifying, especially if they have a close relationship with their partner. They know that pregnancy is itself uncomfortable for the woman, they know that labour is painful, and they know that life is going to change significantly once the baby is born. So it's hardly surprising that even men who are very pleased about the prospect of fatherhood have moments of ambivalence.

Richard's worries are not uncommon:

> 'I wanted a baby more than anything and we had been trying for years, but when it actually happened I felt very scared. Suddenly you have to face the fact that you can't be certain about anything any more. It sounds really petty but you can't even be sure what your wife is going to look like in three months time. I was really looking forward to the birth, but at the same time I kept thinking that we wouldn't be able to have any more quiet Saturday night dinners—just the two of us and a good bottle of wine. There would always be someone else there. I suddenly started worrying about whether I could bear to share Marie with anyone—even our child.'

If a pregnancy is unplanned, however welcome it is, both halves of a couple need time to adjust to the idea.

Going it alone

There are currently over one million lone-parent families in the UK. One family in seven is a single-parent family at any one time and it has been estimated that a third of all children will, at some time, spend a period of time living in a one-parent family.[11]

It is undeniably more difficult to have and raise a child without the support of a partner. This is because society organizes on the assumption that the 'normal' family is one where two adults can divide the responsibility for their offspring between them. Only a minority of families share a 'traditional' division of labour where the father earns a wage while the mother looks after the home, but in many cases social life assumes the majority of people do live in this way. Even something as fundamental as the school day assumes that there is a parent at home to care for the child. Taking a child to, and collecting her from, school is impossible for most full-time workers and can create a number of difficulties for working single parents. Single parents may find it more difficult to participate in the day-to-day life of the school too. Increasingly schools expect parents to play a role in the formal education of their child.

This is something that nearly every parent wants to do, but it takes time—something which a working single mother has in very short supply, as Sue, aged 31, points out.

> 'I was horrified when I was called in to see my daughter's teacher because Jenny was behind with her reading. At the parent's evening they had said that we should spend half an hour each evening reading with our kids because there wasn't time to do individual reading aloud in class—but there was no way I could do it every night.
>
> 'I have two other little ones and by the time I'm in from work and I've sorted out their tea and got them bathed and heard all about what they've been up to it's bed time. To be honest, I'm desperate to get them into bed so that I can get on with the cleaning and washing.
>
> 'Jenny's teacher made it seem like I didn't care. She gave me this long lecture on how important it was for children to learn basic skills. I nearly hit the roof. I don't need to be told how important reading is. I've always loved books. I need to be told how I can fit 28 hours into every day.
>
> 'Anyway, if it's supposed to be down to parents to do reading practice, how are kids whose parents aren't very good at reading supposed to cope—or the kids whose parents really don't care, for that matter.'

Lone parenting is difficult because a lone parent has to shoulder the responsibilities of two, a task that requires a super-human effort.

The difficulties of raising a child single-handed often mean that it is impossible for single mothers to take on the additional responsibility of a full-time job outside the home. This means that single-parents are more likely to experience economic hardship and are often dependent on state benefits.

Absent parents

Absent parents are expected, by the state, to take some responsibility for their children. In the UK, the Child Support Agency (CSA), a new section of the Department of Social Security, has been established to track absent parents and ensure that they make appropriate financial contributions to the upbringing of their children.

From its inception the CSA has been swamped in controversy. Its aims have been supported by some single-parents' organizations such as the National Council for One Parent Families, but other parents groups have opposed its intrusion into what they see as private family relations.

The agency assumes that single women receiving state benefits should be prepared to name the father of their child, so that he may be located by the CSA who will determine how much he should contribute towards maintenance, and ensure that this is paid.

Whilst some women welcome financial support from the father of their child—even if it is unwillingly given, others resent continued contact with a man with whom they had little or no meaningful relationship. Some believe it undermines their independence.

Whatever a woman's individual views on the CSA, if she is claiming any welfare benefits such as income support, family credit, or disability working allowance, she will be expected to provide details of the 'absent parent' including his name, address, and workplace details. If this information is not provided she may lose a proportion of the state benefits she receives.

Of course, if a woman claims she does not know the name of her child's father there is little the Child Support Agency can do to prove otherwise.

The decisions to continue with the pregnancy and to raise her child is the most life-altering choice a woman with an unplanned pregnancy can make. It takes a rapid mental adjustment to new circumstances, but if she is happy about the prospect of motherhood the rewards are unrivalled.

References

1. Report of the RCOG Working Party on Unplanned Pregnancy (1991). Royal College of Obstetricians and Gynaecologists, London.
2. Central Statistical Office (1995). *Social Trends* 25th edn. HMSO, London.
3. See Davies, J., Berger, B., and Carlson, A. (1993). *The family: is it just another lifestyle choice?* Institute of Economic Affairs Health and Welfare Unit, London, *and* Dennis, N. and Erdos, G. (1992). *Families without fatherhood.* Institute of Economic Affairs Health and Welfare Unit, London.
4. Duin, N. and Sutcliffe, J. (1992). *A history of medicine*, pp. 114–15. Simon and Schuster, ??
5. Fourth Report of the Health Committee (1991). *Maternity services: preconception, vol 1.* HMSO, London.
6. Jacqueline Vincent Priya (1992). *Birth traditions and modern pregnancy care.* Element, Shaftesbury.

7. Correy, J.F., *et al.* (1991). Use of prescription drugs in the first trimester and congenital malformations. *Australian and New Zealand Journal of Obstetrics and Gynaecology,* **31**:4, 340–44.

8. Newcomb, W.W., *et al.* (1991). Reproduction in the older gravida. *The Journal of Reproductive Medicine,* **36,** 839–45.

9. Haskey, J. (1994). Estimated numbers of one-parent families and their prevalence in Great Britain in 1991. *Population Trends,* 78, Winter 1994.

10. Data from Robert G. Edwards (ed.) (1993). *Preconception and preimplantation diagnosis of human genetic disease.* Cambridge University Press, Cambridge.

11. Bradshaw, J. and Millar, J. (1991). *Lone parent families in the UK.* Department of Social Services Research Report no. 6. HMSO, London.

Afterword: the right decision?

Whatever decision a woman takes about an unplanned pregnancy, she is sure to wonder what would have happened if her decision had been different. A woman who has chosen an abortion may some- times wish she had continued with the pregnancy and had raised her child. She may wonder what it would have looked like and how she would have matched up to the responsibilities of motherhood. A woman who has given up her child for adoption may have moments when she feels cheated of motherhood, and the woman who has cho- sen to have and raise her child may go through times when she feels bitter about the opportunities which motherhood has excluded her from.

These doubts and regrets do not mean that the wrong decision was taken.

Most of the important decisions that we take are far from clear cut and we often tease ourselves with fantasies about what might have been if we had acted differently or followed another path. This is true of all manner of situations which are important to us. One woman may relive time and time again her decision to change her job, another woman will constantly journey back to the day she left her husband. Yet another may be haunted by a decision not taken: per- haps the chance to emigrate, or to go to college, or to move house.

Few of us have the self-confidence and assuredness never to look back to the past. So it is no wonder that when our past holds a deci- sion about an issue as significant as a pregnancy we constantly drag it from the shadows of yesterday and hold it up to be scrutinized anew. However, when we do this we often look at the old decision in the light of our current circumstances, which may be very different from the time when the original decision was made. This may lead us to think that faced with the same decision again we would make a different choice. And so we might. But that still does not mean that the decision we made before was wrong.

Every woman who experiences an unplanned pregnancy faces a crisis. But the crisis does not have to turn into a disaster. If a woman is able to grasp her situation and take control of it she can still turn the course of her life.

It takes great confidence to draw a line under an incident, to place it firmly in the past, to draw confidence from the experience and to start out again. But as Oscar Wilde wrote in 1897: 'To regret one's own experience is to arrest one's own development.'

Life moves on, we don't have time to stand still.

Appendix: useful addresses

Adoption and foster care

National Foster Care Association,
Francis House
Francis Street
London SW1 1RQ
Tel. 0171 407 8800

National Organisation for the Counselling of Adoptees and their Parents (NORCAP)
3 New High Street
Headington
Oxford OX3 7AJ
Tel. 01865 750 0554

British Agencies for Adoption and Fostering
11 Southwark Street
London SE1 1RQ

Scottish Adoption Advice Service
16 Sandyford Place
Glasgow G3 7NB
Tel. 0141 339 0772
Information and advice about adoption and fostering

Natural Parents' Support Group
10 Alandale Crescent
Garforth
Leeds LS25 1DH
Support for 'birth parents'

Post-Adoption Centre
8 Torriano Mews
Torriano Avenue
London NW5 2RZ
Tel. 0171 284 0555
Support for 'birth parents' and those who have been adopted.

Abortion and contraception

Family Planning Association
27–35 Mortimer Street
London W1N 7RJ
Tel. 0171 636 7866
Information on contraceptive methods and services. Helpline from
10am to 5pm weekdays.

Brook Advisory Centres
165 Gray's Inn Rd
London WC1X 8UD
Tel. 0171 833 8488
Information on contraception and sexual health for young people

Brook Advisory Helpline
Tel. 0171 713 9000
Young person's helpline for contraceptive advice

British Pregnancy Advisory Service (BPAS)
Austy Manor
Wooton Wawen
Solihull
W. Midlands B95 6BX
Tel. 01564 793255
National network of clinics offering pregnancy testing, contraceptive
and abortion advice, counselling, and services.

Marie Stopes Clinics
114 Whitfield Street
London W1P 6BE
Tel. 0171 388 0662
Offers pregnancy testing, contraceptive and abortion advice, coun-
selling, and services. Clinics in London, Leeds, and Manchester

Pregnancy Advisory Service (PAS)
11–13 Charlotte Street
London W1P 1HD
Tel. 0171 637 8962
Offers pregnancy testing, contraceptive and abortion advice, coun-
selling, and services. Clinics in London.

Birth Control Trust
16 Mortimer Street
London W1N 7RD
Tel. 0171 580 9360
Information for professionals on abortion and reproductive health care issues.

Post Abortion Counselling Service
340 Westbourne Park Road
London W11 1EQ
Tel. 0171 221 9631
Advice and counselling following abortion.

Sexual health

National AIDS Helpline
Tel. 0800 567 123
Information about HIV and AIDS

Positively Women
5 Sebastian Street
London EC1V 0HE
Helpline 0171 490 5515
Support for HIV positive women or those with HIV positive partners

Choosing motherhood

National Childbirth Trust
Alexander House
Oldham Terrace
London W3 6NH
Tel. 0181 992 8637
Information and advice about childbirth, breast feeding, etc.

National Council for One Parent Families
255 Kentish Town Road
London NW5 2LX
Tel. 0171 267 1361
Information and advice on benefits, housing, and legal matters.

Maternity Alliance
15 Britannia Street
London WC1X 9JP
Tel. 0171 837 1265
Information about rights and services.

Citizens' Advice Bureaux (CAB)
Details of your local CAB will be in the telephone directory.

Department of Social Security
Helpline for benefits information
Tel. 0800 666 555
Confidential advice on benefits.

Gingerbread
35 Wellington Street
London WC2B 5AU
Tel. 0171 240 0953
Self-help groups for single-parent families.

Lifeline
1st Floor
Ruskin Building
191 Corporation Street
Birmingham
Tel. 0121 233 1641

LIFE
Life House
1a Newbold Terrace
Leamington Spa
Warwickshire CV32 4EA
Tel. 01926 421587/311667
Organizations which offer practical help and advice with continuing the pregnancy—do not provide information on abortion.

Scottish Council for Single Parents
13 Gayfield Square
Edinburgh EH1 3N
Tel. 0131 556 3899
Information on advice for single parents.

Relationship support

Relate—Marriage Guidance
Herbert Gray Colege
Little Church Street
Rugby
Warwickshire CV21 3AP
Tel. 01788 573241

National Association of Mediation and Family Conciliation Services
Shaftesbury Centre
Percy Street
Swindon
Wiltshire SN2 2AZ
Tel. 01793 514055

Family Mediators Association
The Old House
Rectory Gardens
Henbury
Bristol BS10 7AQ
Tel. 01272 500140

Northern Ireland

Ulster Pregnancy Advisory Association
719a Lisburn Road,
Belfast 9
Tel. 01232 381345

Northern Ireland Family Planning Association
113 College Street
Belfast BT7 1HP
Tel. 01232 325 488
Counselling, advice, and information about contraception and abortion.

Belfast Brook Advisory Centre
29A North Street
Belfast BT1 1NA
Tel. 01232 328866
Counselling, advice, and information about contraception for young people.

Ireland

Irish Family Planning Association
5–7 Cathal Brugha Street
Dublin 1
Tel. Dublin 728051/682420

Dublin Well Woman Centre
35 Lower Liffey Street
Dublin 1
Tel. Dublin 728051
or
73 Lower Leeson Street
Dublin 2
Tel. Dublin 610083
Advice on family planning.

Index